ARNICA

How this wonderful plant can be used to ease
both external wounds and mental stress; together
with details of a dozen other homoeopathic
remedies for treating such minor mishaps as
bruises, cuts, sprains, insect bites and headaches.

D0488737

ARNICA
The Amazing Healer

and a Dozen Other Homoeopathic Remedies
for Aches, Pains and Strains

by

A.C. Gordon Ross, M.B., Ch.B., M.F. Hom.

THORSONS PUBLISHERS LIMITED
Wellingborough, Northamptonshire

First published 1977

© THORSONS PUBLISHERS LIMITED 1977

ISBN 0 7225 0374 1

Filmset by Specalised Offset Services Ltd., Liverpool and printed and bound in Great Britain by Weatherby Woolnough, Wellingborough, Northamptonshire.

CONTENTS

For Sheila and Hugh

INTRODUCTION

Whilst it is true that herbalists have a long list of herbs with a reputation for helping injuries, the only ones homoeopaths are sure of are the tried and true favourites; those which have proved their worth time and time again for nearly two hundred years.

Homoeopathy is not fringe medicine. It has been accepted, albeit reluctantly, by the National Health Service, and we have our own hospitals and the Faculty of Homoeopathy, which is empowered to set examinations and award degrees.

This book is, however, in no sense a textbook. I have tried to write it in a cheerful spirit, free from medical jargon, in the hope that it will give thoughtful people some idea how they can cope with minor injuries, and thus save the doctor's time, with the aid of simple and safe medicines kept in the home.

To fix in mind certain points about the remedies used, I have incorporated a number of personal anecdotes and tales which have been with me these many years, and which I hope will have a bearing on each case, and which will not be regarded as too frivolous by the serious-minded reader.

Homoeopathy offers anyone with a rudimentary knowledge of nursing a convenient, safe and cheap method of helping others quickly to get over such minor mishaps as bruises, cuts, sprains, insect bites, sciaticas and headaches without recourse to the family physician.

All that is required is a stock of our injury medicines – the so-called vulneraries – *Arnica, Bellis, Calendula, Hypericum, Ruta, Symphytum, Urtica Urens,* and a few less familiar ones. They can be stocked, away from bright light, in tincture form, or as powders or pills, or as ointments, and they will keep their healing properties almost indefinitely. They are absolutely safe, with none of the side effects which are the bugbear of many modern drugs.

If by chance they do no good they can do no harm, and with our injury remedies the administrator has the enormous satisfaction of seeing a cut dry up and heal (with *Calendula*) in a remarkably short space of time. With *Arnica,* he can see a bruise disappear overnight, with *Urtica* he can see a superficial burn resolve, and not go to blistering tenderness; while with *Ledum* a punctured wound is soon forgotten.

Field-Marshall Viscount Wavell compiled a much praised anthology of poems which was published in 1944 entitled *Other Men's Flowers.* His title was borrowed from Montaigne: '*I have gathered a posie of other men's flowers and nothing but the thread that binds them is my own.*' Most of our homoeopathic injury remedies come from plants, flowers or weeds, and they are bound together in this book for the benefit of those who want to understand.

We must not run away with the idea that Homoeopathy is but an extension of the ancient herbal lore. Homoeopaths can make their medicines not only from plants, but from trees, minerals, snake venoms, macerated insects, the juice of the cuttle fish, and so forth; and they make them potent and harmless by their special method of fragmentation. A method, in fact, that materially-minded scientists used to scoff at, because we could offer them no proof that our special potentization process of succussion had left any trace of the original material in the ultimate product!

Though brought up in a homoeopathic family, I used to worry about those infinitesimal doses, and about the criticism levelled against them by my medical student friends. Surely by dilution, one made a solution weaker and not stronger, until I realized it was the succussion that released the hidden energy in the solution.

When I asked my professor of Organic Chemistry, John Reed, about this he pointed out a passage in his *Text Book of Organic Chemistry*. He was writing about *calciferol* (Vitamin D) and its extreme potency. He wrote: 'One part in more than two thousand millions produces a detectable physiological effect on a rat.'

TESTED ON HUMAN BEINGS

Homoeopaths keep careful records of all their patients, and of the results obtained by potentized medicines. They have all been tested on healthy human beings, not on the lesser animals like dogs, rabbits, rats, or mice. They have been doing this for nearly two hundred years, so there has grown up an enormous accumulation of data, which makes the homoeopath confident about his medicines. He gets to know them as he knows his children, and he is confident that if he finds the similimum, he will get a good result, for the philosophy behind this depends on a principle – *Similia Similibus Curantur* – like cures like. Dr Samuel Hahnemann put forward the fundamental principle that if a single drug is given in disease which can produce similar symptoms in a healthy person, that will bring him back to health, for he understood disease as dis-ease, or disharmony. This is Homoeopathy.

Dr Samuel Hahnemann came from Meissen in what is now East Germany, where his father was a porcelain-painter. I can recollect going to an auction sale at Rosneath Castle which was being sold up with contents after the death of Princess Louise, Duchess of Argyll. There was a tea set of delicate Meissen china: I was not allowed to bid for it for the cups had no handles! It went for £2, and I have often thought they might have been painted by Hahnemann senior.

Samuel's dates were 1755-1843 – a long time to live in those rumbustious times. He was a clever lad, industrious like all Germans, a master of languages, chemistry and medicine.

He got fed up with the poly-pharmacy prevalent at the time, and when translating *Cullen's Materia Medica* – Cullen was an Edinburgh professor – Hahnemann was struck with the idea of experimenting on himself with Quinine (*Cinchona* bark). It was given for the ague and malarial fevers, and Hahnemann found that small quantities of the bark brought on symptoms of the ague in himself – a robust and healthy man. The year before he had noticed that mercury – given for syphilis – brought on mercurial fever, a fever which in some ways resembled the disease. (See *Homoeopathy* by G.R. Mitchell and published by W.H. Allen 1975).

This was Hahnemann's fundamental discovery: that likes should be treated by likes. An old idea, revived by him and made practical by his method of giving minute doses of the medicines, diluted and shaken up. The result of practical experience.

It matters not if drops or grains are given, or administered in infinitesimal fractions of the substance, if such medicines can produce the symptoms in the healthy, they will help the sick.

Now, the injury remedies are peculiar in that one does not require to know all about a patient to administer them with confidence. It is quite obvious if someone in the household gets a cut, bite, insect sting or a burn, and if this book is read or kept for reference, and provided they have the medicines handy, anyone can do a first rate first-aid job.

In an article entitled *Homoeopathy on the High Seas* which I wrote for *The Nautical Magazine*, I suggested that small fishing boats, oil-rigs, and trawlers – often far from medical aid – should carry a handy case of our injury medicines, which the Captain could administer if say a marline-spike dropped on a sailor's bare toes, or if a crewman fell down the hold, or burnt himself in the gallery. The suggestion was taken up by some enterprising sailors.

Of course, some pedants will argue that this is not true homoeopathy, where each case has to be decided on strict individualization, where we must find out all we can about the patient, about his family background, his likes and dislikes, his reactions to various types of food, his reactions to heat and cold, his history of previous illness.

That is all very well when we are dealing with a gastric haemorrhage, a case of pneumonia, or suspected appendicitis, or a sudden fever. These are serious conditions, quite outside the scope of injury medicines, and they require expert handling.

Another may criticize this book because he will say it is bad homoeopathy – merely routine prescribing. For instance, he may ask why I suggest *Ruta* as the homoeopathic medicine for sprained ankles; arguing that if the patient says he feels the pain easier if he gets up and hops about then surely he should be given *Rhus Toxicodendron*.

That is what we call a modality. Modality is a clumsy, old-fashioned word meaning 'the state or condition in respect of mode or manner or modifying influences'. Our text books are full of modalities, ameliorations and aggravations, which help us to choose the matching drug.

For instance, the outstanding modality or modifying influence of *Rhus Toxicodendron* is that the patient feels better by moving about – not what one would expect with a sprained ankle! Patients who react best to *Ledum* are cold creatures with a lack of animal heat; but the peculiarity about *Ledum* is that they are always worse with the heat of the bed, and if they have gout or rheumatism in their lower extremities they like nothing better than to ease them by sticking them in a tub of cold water. The opposite modality to moving about – wants to lie still – is a good indication for *Bryonia,* which does well with pneumonias, pleurisies, and a certain type of rheumatism which has the feature that the pains affect the right side of the body.

Each remedy has its own modality. As one would expect, after a bruise or a blow, *Arnica* is worse for the least touch on the tender part, and the patient feels better for lying down, possibly to get over the initial shock.

I had the honour of helping a German lady revise *Boericke* for a new official German edition of that great Repertory, or storehouse, of homoeopathic information. I must confess, however, that I thought some of the modalities listed in the original American edition were a bit silly. For instance, for *Hypericum* – worse in cold, dampness, in a fog, in close room, least exposure, touch. Better, bending head backwards. Then again, for *Urtica Urens* – worse from snow-air, water, cool moist air, touch. Finally, for *Calendula* – worse in damp, heavy cloudy weather.

Those modalities are repeated in the new German edition, but it is difficult to see how they can help in the choosing of the remedy. I always feel worse in damp heavy cloudy weather, especially if I have a golf match arranged!

TWO COMMON COMPLAINTS

Although not strictly a wound injury, there will be included in this book two very common complaints – lumbago and sciatica – with examples of how we use the modalities to choose the matching remedy. Both conditions seem commoner than ever today, and on several occasions I have been called out on a Saturday afternoon – not the best of times to trouble the doctor – to large houses in the suburbs, where the lawn-mower is standing abandoned on the half-cut lawn. The owner of the house – usually a prosperous hard-working business man – has put in a hard week sitting at a desk, and on his day off, his unwise wife has insisted he cut the grass. As Shakespeare wrote in *All's Well that Ends Well*: 'I am no great Nebuchadnezzar sir, I have not much skill in grass.'

The unfortuante suburbanite – if he was not of the homoeopathic persuasion, would be sent to hospital with suspected coronary thrombosis, or it that was not confirmed, would be sent up to the orthopaedic department to be examined for a possible slipped disc, and would wait patiently for his x-ray.

This has happened several times in my practice, but occasionally if the homoeopath gets there in time, he can alleviate the pain in a matter of hours, and the business man will be back at his desk the following week wondering what all the fuss was about.

What I am trying to do here is to impress upon those interested, the simplicity, the convenience, the satisfaction, a wife could get if she had a few of our well-proved medicines in the house. Then she would put her husband to bed, give him a medicine which she knew could do him no harm if it did not do any good, then call her doctor next day if he had not improved.

I have met with such occasions several times in the course of my practice and those who could give *Aconite* or *Arnica* at once staved off an emergency.

The great Mrs Beeton – who set me on the road to acquiring old cook books many a year ago – wrote *Mrs Beeton's Household Management* before she was fifty. In it she had a good word for *Arnica*: 'tincture of *Arnica*, in the proportion of a teaspoonful to 2 oz. of water is useful in sprains and contusions.'

What a marvellous woman she must have been! She knew the surest way to a man's heart was through his stomach, and she could administer to him when he was bruised. She even knew how to make *Potage Chantilly*.

A 'SIMPLE' DOCTOR
An ancient name for herbal remedies was simples, meaning: 'with nothing added; considered, or taken by itself.' The word brings to mind a story told by J.G. Lockhart (1794-1854) in his biography of Sir Walter Scott. Sir Walter was in England on a visit, and had occasion to call on the services of the local doctor for his coachman. To his amazement he recognized the man as one who started life as a blacksmith in the Borders, and who later became a veterinary surgeon, then progressed to being a doctor.

Scott quizzed the man about his practice, asking him how he did. He was told: 'Sir, my practice is vera sure and orthodox. I depend entirely on two simples.'

'And what may their names be?'

'I'll tell your Honour, ma twa simples are just

Laudamy and Calamy.'

'But John, do you never happen to kill your patients?'

'Kill? Oh ay, maybe sae! Whiles they die and whiles no; but it's the will o' Providence. Onyhow your Honour it wad be long before it makes up for Flodden!'

I like to tell this story to my former medical student friends who took the road to England and made their fortunes in Harley Street and elsewhere, using all modifications of modern science to help – or hinder – their patients' recovery. Simples were perhaps too simple, but they did not commit the doctors to using some of our modern drugs, such as *Thalidomide* and *Eraldin,* the side-effects of which have now become evident, and which have cost, and yet may cost, the highly respectable and famous companies making the drugs enormous sums in compensation.

Homoeopathy has never been popular with the great pharmaceutical manufacturers, who thrive on the varied and ingenious skills of their brilliant organic chemists, who think out new compounds from Carbon, Hydrogen, Oxygen and Nitrogen, to bring out new synthetic drugs, which bring increased profits to the shareholders.

They try them out on the lesser animals – a thing we homoeopaths never do. Perhaps they forget that wise old adage that we interfere with Nature at our peril. We can only hope in years to come that their popular birth pills will not cause damage to the young mothers taking them at the moment.

All suppression is anathema to homoeopaths,

and we think to interfere with the hormone balance in a woman's delicate chemical make-up is bound to lead to trouble, sooner or later.

Perhaps this idea of no suppression is why I gave up carrying a thermometer. Apart from the fact that I was forever breaking them, I realized that a temperature was one of nature's methods of fighting disease. Antipyretics like *Aspirin* merely prolong illness. A persistent temperature in the very old or very young is a different story.

There was a time in my practice when I had the privilege of looking after many worthy farmers and their families. The majority were very good patients, and they even consulted me about their animals: mastitis in cows and so forth. The only drawback was that they were loath to pay their accounts.

One Saturday a farmer's wife 'phoned demanding an urgent visit to see her sick husband. As it was some dozen miles out in the country I suggested I might come on Sunday.

'No, doctor please come today, for Jock has a high temperature.'

'How do you know he has a high temperature?'

'I took it on the dairy thermometer, and it has gone up to cheese.'

He had a 'flu attack and six powders of *Gelsemium* put him right in forty-eight hours.

To sum up, in homoeopathy we treat the patient and not the disease. That is what Dr Margery Blackie meant when she called her fine book *The Patient Not the Cure* (Macdonald and Janes, 1975). A clever title.

In a way an exception to this fundamental

principle is found in most of our wound remedies, where we are treating some external misfortune, and not an inward ill.

> He jests at scars, that never felt a wound.
> But soft! what light through yonder window
>   breaks?
> It is the East, and Juliet is the sun.

If it is not too fanciful we could parody the last line of this famous quotation, imagining the east to be Meissen and changing the name Juliet to Hahnemann!

CHAPTER ONE

ARNICA MONTANA

Arnica Montana, Mountain Arnica, has come down to us from domestic practice. The plant has many names, Leopard's Bane, Mountain Tobacco, Panacea Laprosum, Fall-Kraut (fall-herb), Mountain Daisy. It got its German name (fall-kraut) from the well-known observation that if a sheep sustained a fall on the hill-side, it would nibble the plant, if available.

Arnica belongs to that great botanical family of the Natural Order Composite, which includes among the family, besides *Arnica, Calendula* and *Bellis Perennis*. This trio is regarded by homoeopaths as the principal wound medicine; the other two will be considered in due course.

In *Arnica* we use a tincture of the whole fresh plant, and sometimes a tincture made from the root.

Arnica has bright chrome-yellow flowers, which sometimes reach a height of nearly two feet, rising from a rosette of leaves; dark on the top, but lighter in colour underneath. The root is woody, with a number of small radicles. When macerated it has a peculiar odour, not unlike apples, and has an astringent taste.

The mother tincture is prepared from root, flowers and leaves, but one must get rid of the eggs of the *Arnica* parasitical fly, which feeds on the plant (Dr D.M. Gibson, *Arnica: a Study*, B.H.J. dated 3 July 1972).

It is interesting that Mrs C.F. Leyel says that *Arnica* is diuretic, discutient and stimulant. She is writing from the point of view of a herbalist. Discutient is an old-fashioned word meaning 'Having the quality of dissipating morbid matters.' She does not say anything about *Arnica*'s undoubted value in getting rid of bruises of all kinds, though perhaps discutient covers this action of the plant. (Mrs C.F. Leyel, *Compassionate Herbs* Faber and Faber, 1946).

Dr Gibson says that *Arnica* has a marked affinity with blood vessels, statis, and finally increased permeability, which confirms this finding.

A long time ago, one of my patients, new to Homoeopathy, asked me if it was true we had a panacea for all the ills to which flesh is heir. I am afraid I was a bit hard on the poor man. I told him how we treated the patient and not the disease; and I had many devastating things to say about panaceas, and how the fairground charlatans selling nostrums guaranteed to cure baldness, boils, headaches, skin disorders, and infertility brought herbal lore into disrepute.

After he had gone I looked up panacea in the dictionary to get the exact definition: 'A universal medicine, a healing plant vaguely indicated.'

Then I thought: How about *Panacea Lapsorum* – our *Arnica* – was this what he had in mind? By a coincidence I was reading old Dr Tarbell, A.M., M.D., who published a book '*Homoeopathy Simplified, or Domestic Practice Made Easy*. He published this in Boston in 1874. Dr Tarbell listed thirteen complaints for which he gave a tincture of *Arnica* – one part to ten in water. Bed-sores, bites of insects, boils, bunions, burns, chilblains, contusions, corns, carbuncles, dislocations, black eyes, fractures and toothache. Surely that was a better panacea than most in those far-off days, for Dr Tarbell had a very limited range of remedies to choose from?

HAHNEMANN ON ARNICA

Going back to the master, Hahnemann, he has this to say of *Arnica*:

> Hence it is very beneficial, not only in injuries caused by severe contusions and lacerations of the fibres, but also in the most severe wounds by bullets and blunt weapons, in the pains and other ailments consequent on extracting the teeth and other surgical operations, whereby sensitive patients have been violently stretched: as also after dislocations of joints, after setting fractures of bones etc.

(Quoted by Dr M.L. Tyler, *Homoeopathic Drug Pictures*, Health Science Press 1942.)

Arnica is a short-acting remedy – but it is quick in its action. At the age of thirteen, wearing my first-ever pair of long white flannel trousers, I was cycling down to the local tennis club. The trouser leg caught in the cycle chain, and I was thrown off and concussed. Carried home, my mother gave me *Arnica 30,* and I was in bed for a day or two. I kept my face covered with the bed-sheet. My sisters thought it was because I was ashamed of my accident – they said I had been showing off, but in reality it was because my nose felt cold – *Arnica* had this queer symptom.

Many years later when I was the proud father of an only son, the lady of the house, in the early years of Hitler's War, was cooking a meal in the basement kitchen which had a flagstone floor. She put our small son, aged two, into a rocking-chair, while she got on with the business in hand. Excited, perhaps by the succulent smells coming from the stove, Hugh leaned too far forward, and fell out of the chair, hitting his forehead on the floor. The yells brought me from my consulting room on the floor above. Almost at once a swelling appeared on the lad's forehead. He got *Arnica 30*, two powders and a cold compress of *Arnica* tincture was applied to the swelling. Next day he was as right as rain, with only a slight discoloration and tender spot to show where the injury had been. This cleared after forty-eight hours, and he was none the worse.

That is why I have faith in *Arnica* – for a man can only testify according to his own experience, and homoeopaths have access to careful records kept by earnest practitioners over two centuries, and these records show that *Arnica* is the remedy par excellence for sudden blows of all kinds, where the skin is not broken.

If the evidence of experience was accepted by athletic authorities throughout the world, no football or cricket team would be without *Arnica* in its trainer's kit, no boxing manager nor Olympic athlete would be without his *Arnica*. It should be carried by captains of oil-rigs, by small fishing boats, by motorists, and by climbers in the mountains. The question is – how can we prove to the doubters that what we claim for *Arnica Montana* is based on solid fact?

For years I carried powders of *Arnica* in my golf bag, and on one occasion when I was with a golfing party at Nairn they proved of service. One of my older golfing friends – himself a doctor – collapsed at the sixteenth hole with severe chest pains. He had had a coronary thrombosis some years previously, and this was a second one. I got him back to the hotel on the seat on my trolley-cart and put him to bed partly undressed, after *Arnica 30,* given an hour apart. He had instructions to stay there: but he came down to the cocktail-bar by himself before dinner, to apologize for the trouble caused and to stand us all a drink. He said he felt much better. We got him back to bed as quickly as possible. Unfortunately, he suffered another attack in the course of the night, and died in the Inverness Hospital forty-eight hours later.

I have sometimes thought that *Arnica* could be used to prove its worth against a placebo. Dr R. Gibson, a consultant at the Glasgow Homoeopathic Hospital, was the first to suggest in print that this had practical applications, and Dr Anthony Campbell had an article published in *The British Homoeopathic Journal* entitled *Two Pilot Controlled Trials of Arnica Montana* (3 July 1976).

He made an ingenious apparatus to give artificial bruises to the forearm, and used it on students in the London hospitals – some getting *Arnica* and others the placebo. Potencies 30 and 10m were used, but the results were inconclusive, though the higher potency seemed to work better than the lower one.

A blow that is expected has less impact than a

surprise one, like the knock-out blow in boxing. In the same way an electric shock, if anticipated, is less severe than one totally unexpected! Perhaps this undoubted fact should have been taken into account in this interesting experiment.

One area in which *Arnica* does good work is its usefulness for people who have sustained mental blows of all kinds in their domestic life – sudden frights; bad news; unexpected misfortunes; financial or social calamities.

ARNICA BEFORE AND AFTER SURGERY

Dr Margery Blackie says in her book that surgeons like to see her give *Arnica* to patients undergoing surgery, both before and after the operation. In the old days we used to give *Phosphorus* before operations to avoid bronchial complications from open ether or chloroform. I can remember counting out the drops from the ether bottle as we tried to put our patients away. The art of anaesthesia has advanced by leaps and bounds since that time. My choice of expression is perhaps unfortunate, for if we did not use enough ether some tough patients would leap off the operating table; or try to.

Another very useful field for *Arnica* is after tooth extraction. Not very long ago a lady in this town had an impacted wisdom tooth removed. The dentist had an awful job with it, according to my patient, and the result could be seen in the black and blue bruise resulting on her jaw, which soon cleared up with *Arnica 30*.

If there is much bleeding from the socket after a tooth extraction, a lukewarm *Calendula* mouthwash soon puts matters right. This will be dealt with in a subsequent chapter.

In the course of writing this book it suddenly
struck me that the critics of Homoeopathy – and,
alas, there are many – have said that it has made
no appreciable advance in the last hundred
years. This made me think of Dr Tarbell's book
and his thirteen complaints for which he would
have used *Arnica* in 1874 (see page 21).

He had but few medicines to work with. Today
any competent homoeopath knows that for bites
of any insect, or animal, such as a rat or a dog, if
the wound is sensitive to touch, and relieved by
cold poultices, *Ledum* should be thought of before
Arnica. Again today, he would give *Urtica Urens*
(nettles) for first degree burns, *Tamus* (black
bryony) for chilblaims, *Hepar Sulphuris Calcareum*
(Calcium Sulphide) for suppurating boils,
Tarentula Cubensis (the macerated Cuban spider)
for Cabuncles, and *Symphytum* (Comfrey) for
painful injuries to the eye.

There has been a slow accretion of knowledge,
gathered by homoeopaths all over the world,
from notes kept over the years. True, we have
made no dramatic discoveries like antibiotics,
but what we have done is to pin-point the good
points in the old herbal lore, and we have proved
our medicines, herbal and chemical, time and
again.

I was fond of my examiner in Physiology in my
second year at the 'Varsity. He was a Glasgow
man and, considering that I was an elderly
student in this alien east coast air, he let me
down lightly. He asked me how many calories
were in an egg. I had not the least idea so I

answered: 'Two, sir.' 'Ah!' he said, 'That must be one of your Dundee landlady's eggs!'

Many years later when I was a member of the Glasgow Ballad Club, I met his charming wife, who was a poet in her own right, with two poetry books published in the Angus dialect. That Saturday she was limping badly for she had a calcanean spur on her left heel. I gave her six powders of *Calcarea Fluorica,* potency 30. This is Fluoride of Lime, and in a month, at the next meeting of the club, the calcanean spur was gone without the necessity of that tiresome operation through an incision on the medial margin of her foot. That is why the orthodox medical men say we are full of tricks – but our tricks work, and they have been tried time and again.

Only recently I was going through some old copies of *The British Homoeopathic Journal* – a gold-mine of information well worth re-reading – when I came across an article on homoeopathic injury remedies (B.H.J., 4 October 1959). This was the resumé of a discussion which took place at the sixteenth session of the Faculty in March 1959. In the course of this discussion Dr Noel Pratt of Norwich said that out of his last 600 cases about 10% related to some form of injury. Out of 74 cases *Arnica* was the successful remedy in 30, *Ledum* in 14, *Ruta* in 9, *Hypericum* in 8, *Symphytum* in 8, *Calendula* in 3, and *Silicia* in 2.

Now, just as in even the most affectionate families, we have our own favourite children, so in Homoeopathy we have our own favourite remedies.

Bellis Perennis, the common daisy, is missing from Dr Pratt's list, yet it is one of our oldest injury remedies – even bearing its name from Roman times – 'in fields of battle'. Also he seems to have used *Calendula* only thrice although it is one of our best haemostatic remedies; stopping the flow of blood and healing without scarring. Both *Bellis* and *Calendula* will be considered in due course.

Returning again to *Arnica,* the great Dr James Kent writes in his lectures:

> The first stage of an injury, where much bruising has been done, for shocks and concussions, *Arnica* is routine, because it produces states upon the human body like it had been bruised, but you will find it only fits into that one place. *Arnica* should never be used for wounds the way the lay people use it, because if it is used in full strength it may bring on erysipelas.

Erysipelas, the rose fever, like scarlet fever, is rarely encountered today. Both were caused by streptococci. They were serious illnesses half a century ago, before the appearance of the sulpha drugs.

If not applied too strong, nor too often, five drops of 1c potency to a pint of water, the risk of getting a skin reaction from *Arnica* is minimal. If we use if more freely – in pure tincture undiluted – it is a waste of the mercies, as my mother used to say.

In this short study of *Arnica* I have tried to show how this wonderful plant can be used to ease both external wounds and mental blows, and I conclude with another extract from *Meals Medicinal*, a curious but valuable book by W.F. Fernie M.D., published by John Wright in 1905.

By a strange omission *Arnica* is not mentioned, under 'bruises and sprains' and his list includes: Beef, raw (apply); Bladderwrack, seaweed (for old sprains); Cabbage; Caraway poultice (sprains); Lavendar oil (apply); Mace, pounded (apply); Olive oil; Peas, cooked (apply); Rosemary (sprains); Sea-weed – dulse, laver, samphire (sprains); Verjuice of crab apple; Vinegar poultice (apply cold).

Dr Fernie wrote another book *Herbal Simples* first published by John Wright and Sons in 1895. It went into at least three editions, but here again *Arnica* is not mentioned. It would certainly have been of greater service for bruises than any of the items mentioned above.

I have never understood why *Arnica* is not in every household cupboard. It was as familiar to me as Pears Soap in our family home, but unlike Pears Soap, it has never been properly advertised.

NOTES ON DOSAGE

Every household should keep a 4 fl. oz. (100 ml) bottle of 'mother' tincture for use diluted in equal part for external application to bruises of all kinds.

At the same time give *Arnica 30* (one) in pill form every two hours. Continue for four doses.

Keep a stock of pills (5g). They can be used for any age, but very young children should have the pill crushed and given on a wet teaspoon as they are apt to spit out whole pills.

CHAPTER TWO

BELLIS PERENNIS

The humble daisy is the second of our homoeopathic wound remedies, more familiar to most than *Arnica*, but belonging to the same large Natural Order, the Compositae. It gets its Roman name from *Bellis* – 'in fields of battle', and *Perennis* implies that though the rose has but a short summer season, the daisy never dies.

It used to be said that spring has not arrived until a person could put a foot on twelve flowering daisies on the lawn at once – and the more they are trodden on the better they grow. The daisy is known to homoeopaths as the gardener's remedy, for after some unaccustomed gardening a dose or two of *Bellis* gets rid of that muscular stiffness common to week-end gardeners.

Last year I had an enormous crop of daisies on my lawn, and, one fine summer's day, being stuck for an idea how to entertain two small visitors making daisy chains, I presented the two girls with a bucket apiece, and offered them a small reward if they filled each bucket with daisy heads. From them I made daisy whisky.

Chaucer said on rising and seeing daisies on the lawn: 'That blissful sighte, softeneth al my sorwe.'

The flowers and leaves of the daisy are found to afford a considerable quantity of oil and of ammoniacal salts. The root was named *Consolida*

Minima by older physicians, and Fabricius speaks of its effect in curing wounds and contusions. A decoction of the leaves and flowers was given internally and the bruised herb blended with lard was applied externally. 'The leaves stamped do take away bruises and swellings, whereupon it was called in old time bruise wort.' (*Herbal Simples,* W.T. Fernie, M.D., John Wright, 1914).

Being a diminutive plant, with roots to correspond, the daisy, according to the Doctrine of Signatures, was formerly thought to arrest the bodily growth, and its roots, boiled in broth, were given to young puppies so as to keep them of a small size.

Dr Peter Engel says that the conditions that *Bellis* can help are not rare, and include vertigo in the elderly, sprained calf muscles, traumatism of the pelvic organs, and varicose veins during pregnancy that impede walking. Most prominent is the affinity of *Bellis* for the muscular walls of the blood vessels of the toes. He gives an example of an old gardener in his own practice whom he cured of gangrene on the third toe of his right foot with *Bellis* in low potency (3x) five drops to be taken thrice daily. (*Some Remedies from Common Plants*, Dr Peter Engel, British Homoeopathic Journal Vol. 61).

Daisies were said of old to be under the dominion of Venus, and later on they were dedicated to St Margaret of Corona. Therefore they were reputed to be good for the special illnesses of females, which is confirmation of Dr Engel's statement about injury to the pelvic organs and varicose veins. Dr Boericke confirms all of Dr Engel's assertions, though he states that another symptom is itching around scalp and over back, worse from a hot bath, and he also suggests it for crops of boils.

Its main use, however, is for sore joints and stiffness in muscles unaccustomed to use, especially on the left side.

GOOD FOR DUCKINGS

I had a good result with *Bellis* when I happened to have my medical case handy when a small child of about three years old fell into the swimming pool at St Andrew's. There was no danger, for he was pulled out at once, but his yells had to be heard to be believed. Two powders of *Bellis 30* quietened him at once, but his mother was also full of indignation because I had failed to keep adequate watch on her child. She got one powder of *Arnica* to soothe her ruffled feelings. *Bellis* has the symptoms: worse for duckings.

On another occasion when I was but newly qualified I regretted not having my medical case with me. I was fishing in the far north, when a sickly-looking youth from my hotel went off for a swim. Now, our Highland lochs are cold and deep, and the unlucky swimmer caught a chill. That night he had all the appearances of pneumonia – flushed face, quickened breathing, restless and a bronchial cough. Personally I thought we would have to take him to hospital in Inverness fifty miles away, but a wise old retired doctor on holiday in the hotel thought otherwise. He asked me to take a flannelette sheet down to the lochside and soak it in the cold water. This done he wrapped his patient in it, having taken off his pyjamas, and put him between blankets with two hot water bottles. It was before the days of *Penicillin* or the sulpha drugs, and next day he was much better, and down for breakfast two days later.

This incident stuck in my mind for more than fifty years. I used to wonder if perhaps it was not one more example of the homoeopathic principle being proved, for *Similia Similibus Curantur*, or like cures like, stays in the public imagination as 'the hair of the dog'.

Anyone interested in poetry knows of Andrew Young. He wrote a delightful book called *A Prospect of Flowers*. He has this to say about the common daisy: 'Chaucer would approve, for to him it was "The Emperice, and floure of floures alle" Though Burns called it: "Wee, modest, crimson-tipped flow'r".'

The daisy is not modest. Like an impudent juggler who spreads his mat in a crowded street, it spreads its leaf-rossette on the ground, stands on it and defies interference from other plants. How could it be modest when we have named it Daisy – the Eye of Day? But perhaps we were thinking not of an eye that opens, but of an eye that shuts? In the evening 'Daisies button into Buds' (John Clare)

Looking like white pitched tents: in fact, if the crimson tips are for warmth, they are, so to speak, their own tent and fire, and, strangely enough, no flower has reminded poets more of death: I know not why thy beauty should, Remind me of the cold dark grave' (Thomas

Hardy). It ought to be a cheering flower, this *Bellis Perennis* – the Perenially Pretty: 'The constellated flower that never sets' (Shelley) and who ever saw a withered daisy?

Andrew Young in his fine book remarks somewhere that few poets took an interest in botany – but he comes close to doing so himself. He remarks:

> The greater Celandine's milk [our *Chelidonium Matus*] is yellow: it was considered a cure for jaundice. A homoeopathic cure we may say, for Homoeopathy means sympathy, the sympathy in this case, being shown in the likeness of the milk's colour to the patient's. Perhaps it was a homoeopathic cure in the other sense, taken in small doses, for it is bitter milk.

When his book came out I wrote to Andrew Young to tell him that, while he was right about the jaundice, he had gone astray in the meaning of Homoeopathy, which, of course, means like sickness and not sympathy. He sent back a very humble reply, acknowledging his error.

There are great possibilities for poets and romantic writers in a study of herbal lore, and it is interesting and good fun to compare their approach to plants with that of the homoeopath and the herbalist. For instance, knot-grass (*Polygonum Aviculare*), in material doses of the tincture, has been used by us for glandular fever and arterio-sclerosis. I came across it first when making a study of the very numerous grasses to help hay-fever subjects. Like the daisy, knot-grass kept one small. Shakespeare writes of it as 'Hindering knotgrass' due to its reputation for retarding growth.

Then there is a type of fern called Moonwort, (*Botrychium Lunardia*) Culpeper said it is difficult to find for it grows among much grass, but if gathered in moonlight, it has the reputation of being able to open locks. As a herb it was supposed to heal wounds and, when boiled in white wine and made into lotions, it was good for bruises and sprains.

As Andrew Young remarks: 'In Knot Grass and Moonwort, an enterprising burglar had a complete outfit – especially if he knew the virtue of Fern Seed – which was supposed to make one invisible.' surely with these four plants Knotgrass, Daisy, Moonwort, and Fern Seed, the modern detective writer could arm himself with material for a good story.

ACCUMULATED LEGENDS

It is perhaps because of the accumulated legends that linger around herbal literature that our great profession looks askance at our plant remedies.

The reviewer of Dr Blackie's book in *The Field* puts it rather well in a paragraph headed 'Herbal Suspicions'. She is writing about Hahnemann's dictum that the highest ideal of cure is a rapid, gentle and permanent restoration of health.

She says: 'This, surely, is of interest at a time when many feel that a number of cures effected by orthodox allopathic (chemical) medicine are not gentle if rapid, not complete if gentle, and seldom permanent in either case. Why then, since Homoeopathy has existed for nearly two centuries and claimed some remarkable cures, is homoeopathic treatment not more widely sought? ... Partly, perhaps, because it uses plant substances in fairly simple forms in its Materia Medica and because plants, or "herbs" as they are more often called in this context, are regarded with suspicion by many, having been at one time the last resort of the ignorant and superstitious, and lately too often and too dogmatically thrust at us by people whose other eccentricities weaken their credibility.'

In my book *Homoeopathy: An Introductory Guide* (Thorsons) I asked why Homoeopathy, with all its good points – safety, certainty, cheapness, gentleness – has not swept the country and become an integrated part of medical care? The short answer is mass medication, dramatic discoveries such as antibiotics and cortizone, no encouragement from the establishment, or the academics, and bureaucratic control.

NOTES ON DOSAGE

For stiffness and sudden duckings keep a small stock of pills, and give one at night for stiffness and at once for sudden duckings. Use potency 30.

CHAPTER THREE

CALENDULA OFFICINALIS

Calendula is our next wound medicine, prepared from the tall marigold growing wild on non-acid soil. Old Culpeper called the marigold 'The Herb of the Sun'. Like African Daisies (*Mesembryanthemums*) the marigold opens its petals on a sunny morning but closes them on a wet day. It has a peculiar smell, apparently anathema to the eel-worm, and root crops can be protected from this pest by the companion planting of marigolds.

A CURE FOR GOUT

Not many miles from where we live there is a ruined monastery with the remains of a walled herbal garden, which contains nothing now but Bishops' weed and a few marigolds. Bishops' weed gets its name from the fact that the monks cultivated it as a cure for gout, just as they used the marigold as possets and drinks and as a comforter for the heart.

The name *Officinalis* shows the marigold's connection with the holy men, and its uses in medicine go back even earlier than the sixteenth century. It is the homoeopathic remedy excelling all others for open cuts which will heal by first intention without stitching. In the run-of-the-mill working of a practice there are always cuts to be sewn up. Neither my brother nor myself were good needlemen, so we fell into the habit of putting *Calendula* tincture in warm dressings on all our cuts. They nipped a bit at first, but stopped the bleeding quickly, and it was remarkable how *Calendula* closed the cuts up so promptly, and rarely left a scar.

I can recollect a lady who sustained a two inch cut above her left eyebrow. It bled profusely, and looked as if it would need to be stitched, but I had neither needle nor stitching material with me so the hot *Calendula* technique was applied. A year later, when I saw the lady again, the mark was scarcely discernible, but the patient complained that when she raised her eyebrows one went higher than the other – much to the amusement of her friends!

A PRETTY WAITRESS

On another occasion which I well remember – for I had just done the sixth hole-in-one at Dornoch – I went down to the shore with my accountant to watch the bathing. Larking around was a pretty trainee waitress from the hotel with the waiter from our table. The lass trod on a broken lemonade bottle and sustained a nasty cut on the side of her foot. We got her to the hotel – a matter of 200 yards – as quickly as possible, and the cut was cleaned with *Calendula* and a firm bandage applied.

Two years later came the sequel. My accountant friend and I were at another hotel on the West Coast, where we got great attention from the under-manager, including a complimentary bottle of wine on the night of our departure. Such hospitality is unusual in a railway hotel, so when it came to paying the bill I asked why we had received such fine service. Apparently the waiter had progressed in his profession to under-manager, and had married the pretty young girl whose foot had been cut.

As I explained to the smiling fellow, I had always known that *Calendula* knitted the flesh together, but not to that extent!

Calendula cleans as well as knits, and is useful when children scrape their knees from a tumble on gravel paths. Its haemostatic effect is quite remarkable after tooth extraction. No need to plug the empty socket with cotton wool. Ten drops of *Calendula* tincture in half a tumbler of tepid water, makes an admirable non-poisonous mouth wash, most soothing to the patient.

Marigolds are popular all over the country in cottage gardens, and Mrs Leyel says in *Cinque Foil*: 'the name *Calendula* is supposed to derive from the fact that it may be found in bloom somewhere in every calendar month. As a domestic medicine, the marigold is one of the best herbs available to man and it is so easy to grow that no garden should ever be without it. After accidents, for cuts and inflammations of any kind, when the skin has been broken, it would never be wrong to apply it locally, or to take internally a hot decoction of these flowers. (Make with a pint of boiling water to two handfuls of the flowers and leaves.) It promotes healthy granulation, it is a cordial herb, and as such excellent for the heart and circulation.'

BAD CIRCULATION

Incidentally, I can bear out Mrs Leyel's last sentence from personal experience in my own

family circle. My mother-in-law, a grand old
lady who lived with us and died some years ago
at the ripe age of ninety-two, was much bothered
with bad circulation in her feet. They looked
painful and occasionally the skin broke. The old
lady was never without her *Calendula,* both in
tincture and ointment. She said it was the only
thing that kept her on her feet – that and keeping
an eye on her son-in-law!

In John H. Clarke's *Materia Medica* he
mentions *Calendula* as preventing suppuration
and pyaemia, and in some cases of carbuncle it
acts with great promptitude, subduing pain and
fever.

I had a parson once as a patient who was
hoarse. He had the Scottish habit of preaching
forty-minute sermons. At first I tried him with
Arum Triphyllum, known as Jack-in-the-Pulpit,
but it did no good. Then I tried him with Borax
crystals to suck before he started but they went
off the market. *Calendula* was his salvation. He
gargled with a weak solution before ascending
the pulpit, had a swig of water with *Calendula* in it
during his discourse if he felt the hoarseness
coming on, and declared he could go on till
Doomsday which, according to him, was at
hand.

Our next wound medicine to be considered
will be *Hypericum,* (St John's Wort), which always
has had a great homoeopathic reputation in
injury to a nerve which has become irritable and
inflamed.

Although as a rule, we homoeopaths do not
believe in mixing our drugs, Nelson's of London
find a growing demand for *Hypercal* tincture,

which is a mixture of equal parts of Nelson's fresh plant tincture of *Hypericum Perforatum* and *Calendula Officinalis*. They say the remarkable healing and bacteriostatic qualities of *Calendula,* combined with the well known pain-relieving properties of soothing *Hypericum,* produce a most effective application. The fresh flowering wild plants are tinctured with pure alcohol so that the final strength of the finished product in each case consists of two-thirds by volume of natural plant juice.

The resulting very low alcoholic strength permits the application of the undiluted tincture to small cuts and abrasions without undue smarting, and should a second application be necessary, smarting is usually absent.

NOTES ON DOSAGE

As with *Arnica* each household should keep a 4 fl. oz. (100 ml) bottle of 'mother' tincture and use it diluted in equal part in lukewarm water for open cuts and as a mouthwash in cases of sore throats. It is non-poisonous.

Also keep a stock of pills (5g) and give one four hours apart. Use potency 30.

CHAPTER FOUR

HYPERICUM PERFORATUM

Hypericum reigns in solitary state as the only member of the botanical Natural Order *Hypericaceae*.

Perhaps because it was lonely in that isolation, Nelson's have combined it with *Calendula* in the form of *Hypercal* – a logical step for a vulnerary which is gaining in popularity. The word *Hypericum* means 'sub-heather' and yet in my garden the plant does not take kindly to the Ericas.

Herbalists know *Hypericum* as St John's Wort, not to be confused with St John's Herb, or Holy Rope. The plant has short runners, and the flowers have five chrome-yellow pointed petals, twice as long as the five green sepals. It flourishes between July and September, when the bush can be pruned back severely.

As Dr D.M. Gibson wrote in the *B.H.J.* 3 July 1972: 'When crushed, the flowers leaves and stems emit a curious, almost resinous scent. This persists in the mother tincture, prepared from the whole fresh plant. The plant if injured exudes a reddish-brown juice, suggestive of blood which may account for its use as a vulnerary'.

Hypericum has been well proved as the remedy above all others, for injured nerves and for parts rich in nerves.

ABSCESSES AND PAINFUL INJURIES

Like *Calendula*, *Hypericum* can close the lips of wounds, thus avoiding stitching, and it has also the opposite virtue, well expressed by Culpeper more than 300 years ago, that 'It opens obstructions and dissolves swellings'. Hence it should be thought of for abscesses, and for any injury where there is much pain.

I once tried *Hypericum* on a parson who had a persistent dream that his wife had been turned into a witch in a Welsh hat. His second symptom was that he was a martyr to lumbago, and that he had earache – possibly from his badly fitting hearing-aid. Three symptoms – did he have a fourth? Yes! He suffered from dizzy spells. Now all symptoms are covered by *Hypericum,* more or less, but without much result after I had given it to him.

On his next visit I told him the story of a patient who went to his doctor complaining of occasional vertigo. He did not smoke or drink – tobacco and alcohol are common causes – so he had his ears washed out. He was better for a day or two, but the vertigo returned, so he demanded to see a specialist, who did the fenestration operation on his deaf ear. After paying a substantial fee, he was no better, so he returned to the specialist who said he must have a brain tumour and that the prognosis was bad. On his way home he went to his shirtmaker to get him to make two new shirts, size 16 collar.

The shirtmaker said he had put on weight since his last order, and he would like to measure his neck. 'Not at all,' said the customer, 'I am in a hurry. I have been wearing size 16 for years'.

Eventually he was persuaded, and the shirtmaker said, 'Sir, your neck size is 17 – if you are wearing size 16, you are bound to feel giddy and have a ringing in your ears!'.

There was no reaction from my patient to this story – he had not heard it, for his hearing-aid had gone phut, perhaps just as well! Eventually the old chap improved with *Sulphur* in high potency. I should have thought of this sooner, for he hated hot summers and hot baths, and when young had eczema on his legs.

Gerard has this to say regarding *Hypericum*:

The leaves, floures and seeds stamped, and put into a glasse with oile olive, and set in the hot sun for certain weeks together and then strained from these herbs, and the like quantitie of new put in and sunned in like manner, doth make an oile of the colour of blood, which is a most pretious remedie for deep wounds and those that are thorow the body, for the sinues that are prickt, or for any wound made with a venomed weapon.

Gerard wrote this before 1636, when his *Herball* was published.

Dr Margaret Tyler in her *Homoeopathic Drug Pictures* explains that the 'Doctrine of Signatures' was really responsible for the discovery of many common medicines, the idea being that The Almighty had set His seal on substances and plants useful for healing, so that they might be recognized by His suffering children in their need ... And indeed, most of the liver medicines are yellow *Berberis*, *Chelidonium*, and so on, while the remedies that affect the blood especially are red – the salts of *Iron*, *Hypericum*, *Hammamelis*, and others. Dr Tyler wrote pen pictures of 115 drugs and her book is as fresh today as when it came out in 1942. Her father was Sir Henry Tyler, who gave generously to the London Homoeopathic Hospital – now the Royal London Homoeopathic Hospital, due to the Royal Patronage.

BENEFITS OF HYPERICUM

Nothing, however, beats personal experience, so here are two incidents illustrating the benefits of *Hypericum*.

At the age of eighteen I was about to play rugby for the Glasgow Academy against their old rivals The Glasgow High School. On my way to the match the first finger of by left hand got caught in a door of a railway carriage. I played through the match in agony and when I went home my brother, Dr T.D. Ross, in his final year of medicine, put on a *Hypericum* dressing, 10 drops of the tincture in cold water. The dressing was changed twice and next day the pain subsided, though the nail went black. The extravasated blood was let out by boring a hole in the nail with a darning needle, which convinced me that my brother would make his name in his chosen profession, which he did.

The second occasion happened many years later in the dark days of Hitler's war. The husband of a patient – a young chap of twenty-three lost a leg and was invalided out of the Army. His wife phoned one day to say she was thinking of taking him to a psychologist as he kept complaining of pain in the toes of the leg which was not there. I sent him *Hypericum* 30, and after ten days the young wife phoned to say her husband had no more trouble though the depression, often a symptom calling for *Hypericum*, remained with him a long time until he got used to wearing his artificial limb.

Perhaps the best study of *Hypericum* in our literature comes from Dr J.T. Kent whose *Lectures on Homoeopathic Materia Medica* (Boericke and Tafel, Philadelphia 1923) is a volume which should be studied in conjunction with Dr John H. Clarke's *Dictionary of Materia Medica* – a massive work in three volumes.

Dr Kent stated: 'The surgery of Homoeopathy largely involves the use of Arnica, Rhus Toxicendron, Ledum, Staphisagria, Calcarea and Hypericum.' This was written in 1904; nowadays he would add to the list *Calendula, Bellis,* and perhaps *Urtica Urens* and *Ruta*.

NERVE INJURIES

Dr Kent says *Hypericum* and *Ledum* run close together in the kind of injuries for consideration when an injury to a nerve has taken on inflammatory action, or when the finger-ends or toes have been bruised or lacerated, or a nail has been torn off, or when a nerve has become pinched between a hammer and the bone in a blow. When that nerve becomes inflamed and the pain can be traced up along the nerve and is gradually extending towards the body from the injured part with stitching, darting pains coming and going, or shooting up from the region of the injury towards the body, a dangerous condition is coming on. In this condition *Hypericum* is, above all other remedies, to be thought of.

What Dr Kent was thinking of was Tetanus or

Lockjaw, which can occur after an injury to
sentient nerves. The dominant school often given
an anti-tetanus injection almost as a matter of
routine but *Hypericum* can prevent such tragedies
developing, as can *Ledum* or *Cicuta* (water
hemlock). *Hypericum* is also a remedy to be
thought of in such conditions which used to be
called 'railway spine' – any injuries to the
vertebrae, such as the common one in the home,
where the housewife comes down hard on her
fundament when her feet go from her and she
gets severely jarred.

The coccyx in a woman is often injured when a
woman has a difficult birth and she endures low
back pain for years. She may get *Sepia* on her
presenting symptoms, but if the condition does
not clear up, *Hypericum* should be considered.

When I was young I revered the Poet
Laureate, Dr Robert Bridges, who wrote *The
Testament of Beauty*. I also worshipped John
Galsworthy – but both have gone out of fashion
because the verdict of posterity is that both were
sententious prigs. I did not quite believe this of
Robert Bridges, until I came across a remark by
Andrew Young – one of our real genuine English
poets:

> Was Eve (our first Eve) so refined that she would
> have approved of Bridges calling St John's Wort,
> Sinjunwort? As the plant was named after the
> Baptist, about whose feast-day it flowers, he has
> not the authority of the Curate who spoke of the
> gospel according to Sinjun!

(*A Prospect of Flowers*, Andrew Young, Cape,
1945).

A gentle reproof from one of our gentlest of poets.

NOTES ON DOSAGE

Keep in stock a 4 fl. oz. (100 ml) bottle of 'mother' tincture and use diluted in equal part in lukewarm water for injuries such as crushed finger nails and superficial nerves.

Hypercal tincture is a mixture of *Calendula* and *Hypericum* and could also be stocked.

CHAPTER FIVE

LEDUM PALUSTRE

This is an unattractive name for a plant belonging to the *ericaceae* family, of the tribe *rhodoreae*, which includes our *Kalmia Latifolia* (mountain Laurel) and Rhododendron. The name *Ledum* comes from the Greek word *Leoos* – a woollen toga, and it is sometimes called Wild Rosemary, Labrador Tea, or Marsh Tea.

It is a small shrub, resembling a tea plant, and likes to grow in cold climates, but it is found here at high altitudes, growing in peat bogs and on Sphagnum moors. The flowers are in terminal clusters, small and white, on long stalks, while the seeds are many, flat and strap-like. The plant has a bitter taste, and when bruised emits a strong aromatic, oppressive odour, somewhat like hops.

The flowers contain an antiseptic, camphor-like oil, Ledol, which is responsible for the scent, and the mother tincture is prepared from the dried twigs, or from the whole freshly gathered plant. I have derived most of this information from Dr Gibson's pen-picture of the plant (he has written many which are bound to become classics of their kind) given in *Homoeopathy* by Dr D.M. Gibson, M.B., F.R.C.S., April/May 1974.

Thinking of *Ledum* and its two cousins in the family, *Kalmia* and *Rhododendron,* I know they all flourish best in acid soil, and we are not surprised that homoeopaths use all three for rheumatism,

but the rheumatisms of *Kalmia* start from the feet
and work upwards, while a *Ledum* rheumatism
travels downwards, and *Rhododendron* acts best on
the small joints of the extremities.

The dominant school has no appreciation of
the subtle differences we have in our choice of
medicines. For instance, patients requiring *Ledum*
are chilly patients but they are aggravated by
heat, preferring a cold bath to a hot one.
However as this little book is primarily about our
wound healers, we do not need to concern
ourselves too much about these differences
(which take a lost of memorizing, even with a
repertory) and we concentrate here on the role of
Ledum as a wound healer.

AN OUTSTANDING TRIO

Old Dr Nash had the good idea of grouping his
remedies according to their modalities (*Leaders in
Homoeopathic Therapeutics*, E.B. Nash M.D.,
Boericke and Tafel, 1901), and if we were to do
this for our wound remedies, we would find an
outstanding trio in *Arnica, Hypericum,* and *Ledum*.

The feature about *Ledum* is that it is pre-
eminent for punctured wounds of all kinds,
whether caused by a nail piercing the foot, or by
a tack on a ship's deck, or by bites and stings
from the biting midges (*Chirononidae*) or the sand
flies (*Psychodidae*).

Midges are a perfect plague in the West of
Scotland. I well remember on the first day of
Hitler's war I thought it incumbent on me to
remove my sister and her four small children out
of Glasgow. Her husband was building a bridge
in China at the time.

I chose Lochgoilhead, and established them in a small hotel run by a patient. They did not stay more than a few days, for my sister said she would rather be bombed in Glasgow, than see her babies eaten to death by midges!

Incidentally, I had another patient in that remote village who carried on a unique romance with a retired sea-captain at Carrick, some few miles down Loch Goil on the west side. When the tide was coming in, he would write a loving message on a plank of wood and launch it in the loch. Her house was at the water's edge and she would reply on the ebb tide. The romance prospered, as it deserved to do.

Dr Nash remarks: 'In injuries where *Arnica* is best at first, *Ledum* often removes the ecchymoses and discoloration more rapidly and perfectly. He also says that 'for a black eye, from a blow or contusion, there is no remedy to equal *Ledum* in the 200th potency (in powder form) but if there is great pain in the eye ball itself, *Symphytum* (Comfrey) may have to be used'.

TETANUS

The great Dr J.T. Kent makes the dramatic and perhaps dogmatic assertion that, for a punctured wound, if *Ledum* is given at once it will prevent Tetanus. This is a horrible condition, almost as terrifying to the lay public as Rabies. I am fortunate to have no experience of either calamity.

In the homoeopathic literature I can only find one case of recorded treatment. Dr G.H.G. Jahr, in his book *Forty Years' Practice* says that he used *Angustura Vera,* potency 30, of which a teaspoonful every half-hour soon controlled the convulsions. Anti-tetanus serum should be the modern treatment, but here again there is the risk of anaphylactic shock, as in the case quoted by Sir John Weir, to which I will refer later on and where he gave *Aconite*.

Homoeopaths are not keen on vaccinations or injections of any kind, perhaps because the majority of our patients in a homoeopathic practice are of the allergic type, whose reason for trying homoeopathy in the first instance, was because our remedies have the reputation of causing no adverse reactions.

Time and again a mother has said when bringing an asthmatic or eczematous child: 'Doctor, he has never been right since being vaccinated against smallpox as a baby.' The same story is told – but not so often – about injections against measles and whooping cough in the treatment of the young.

Vaccination is required for passport regulations in persons going abroad, just as they require cholera, yellow fever, and anti-typhoid injections, but most requiring those were adults who were well used to the routine over the years. No doubt if a patient demanded anti-tentanus serum or toxoid, arrangements would be made for this to be given, but only as a last resort.

Sitting now on the side lines, I am inclined to think that the fear of Rabies in this country is perhaps a little overdone and poses a problem to all animal lovers. On the Continent they have learned to live with it, and it is foolish to assume that if Rabies does reach Britain, every bite from a dog or nip from a cat, means Rabies and that the outcome will be fatal.

We homoeopaths have *Hydrophobinum*, potentized from *Lyssin* – the saliva of a rabid dog. It is said to be a specific for Hydrophobia, with the modality that the patient is made worse by the sound or sight of running water and fears he is going mad. I have never used it in my practice.

NOTES ON DOSAGE

Keep a 5g stock of pills, and give one every four hours for two days to remove discoloration following a bad bruise. Use potency 30.

CHAPTER SIX

RUTA GRAVEOLENS

Ruta is the familiar Rue, from the natural order *Rutaceae*, which includes *Citrus Linonum*, *Jaborandi* and *Angustura Vera*. We use a tincture of the whole plant while fresh.

It is of very ancient reputation in medicine – 'The Herb of Grace' – 'The Herb of Repentance' – and is one of the earliest of our vulneraries, helping in injuries not only of the soft parts, but of the bones and periosteum (the periosteum is the tough fibrous sheath surrounding bone).

In Hahnemann's *Materia Media Pura* he writes: 'This powerful plant, hitherto almost only employed in haphazard fashion by common folk as a domestic remedy in indeterminate cases, acquires considerable importance from symptoms observed from its administration.' The blind poet John Milton knew the virtué of *Ruta* in one of its main fields of action – to help eye strain and injuries to the eye – when he recommended 'Euphrasie and Rue to clear his visual ray.' ...

Teste wrote: 'Even in our own time the Roman ladies imagine that the most odoriferous flowers may be left in their rooms without the least danger provided a bush of garden Rue be amongst them'. Shakespeare knew this too. He had a great interest in matters medical, and would have made a good doctor:

For you there's Rosemary and Rue, these keep seeming and savour all the winter long.
(*The Winter's Tale*.)

TWISTED ANKLE

One of the best results I had with *Ruta* has stuck in my mind these many years. This was with a young woman who had gained no small reputation in the West of Scotland as a tennis player of great potential. I had looked after her parents from time to time, but I had never had occasion to meet her, she was an uppity miss at a fancy school in the South before she blossomed out.

She consulted me in breathless fashion late one afternoon, because she had twisted her right ankle, which was badly swollen. I asked her if this had occurred while playing tennis? 'Indeed not,' she said, 'I turned my ankle on the stair while sliding down a banister.' She must have been twenty-two at this time, very soigné and reticent, and a bit nervous, for she was not used to doctors – so she said.

I gave her *Ruta,* six powders of potency 30c, and I put a cold compress of *Ruta* mother tincture on her swollen ankle. She was back on the tennis courts within a week and got into the final of the women's doubles.

In this instance I had to decide between *Arnica, Ruta,* or *Rhus Toxicodendron. Ruta* won because the modality was that she said she was worse lying down. *Rhus* has that too, but she was better resting than moving about. This precluded *Rhus* and also *Arnica,* which has the modality worse from touch and the least motion, and in any case *Ruta* has a special affinity for the flexor tendons.

To quote from John H. Clarke's *Dictionary of Materia Medica* again:

The vulnerary remedies indicate in symptoms of their provings, the peculiar form of injuries for which Hahnemann's provings are adapted. There are the sprained pains of *Rhus Toxicodendron,* the bruised pains of *Arnica* (in skin and muscles).

Ruta also has the bruised pains, but these are more particularly manifest in bones. Ruta is one of the chief remedies for injured bones. ...

I think this is a bit misleading, for with an injury like a sprained ankle it is the tendons that are stretched and the bones rarely injured. This is the kind of situation where experience is of value.

One of the best books ever written about homoeopathy is *An Introduction to the Principles and Practice of Homoeopathy* by Dr Charles E. Wheeler. The earnest student reading that very fine writer, might think *Rhus Toxicodendron* was the remedy – especially if he knew Dr Clarke's Comments too – for Wheeler has this to say about Rhus:

Rhus is particularly suitable to affections of joints, tendons and fibrous tissues that are the result of over-strain (over-lifting for instance) or the effects of over-exertion of a group of muscles.

Who am I to set myself up against two of our most revered authorities? But the proof of the pudding is in the eating – and I think *Ruta* did more for the tennis-playing lady than *Rhus* could have done.

WRIST INJURIES

Dr E.B. Nash remarks (somewhat carelessly) that the pains and lameness of *Ruta* seem to have a particular liking for the wrists. Difficult to imagine how one could be lame in the wrist – but he is accurate when he says that *Ruta* does help wrist injuries.

Ruta came into my reckoning when I coped with the old lady's Colles fracture (see next chapter) but at ninety-five I thought the thing to go for was to assist the bones to knit and Symphytum was the obvious choice – she could get *Ruta* later but in her case she did not need it.

> Rue maketh chaste: and eke preserveth sight
> infuseth wit, and putteth fleas to flight ...

During the war six very poor and dirty children were evacuated to my uncle's house in Stirling. He put Rue leaves among the sheets in their beds, in a vain attempt to get rid of fleas and nits in their heads. He was surprised to find the leaves irritated their skins, but he did not know his Gerard's *Herball*. Gerard wrote: 'The wild Rue venometh the hands that touch it, and will also infect the face'.

My uncle called me to cope with the nits in their hair and all I could think of was to shampoo the heads with petrol, which did the trick. I had advised him to use *Staphisagria* – it got the name as an exterminator of head lice – but the Glasgow lice were too much for even *Staphisagria* in the case of the Glasgow kids.

NOTES ON DOSAGE

Keep a 5g stock of pills and give one every four hours for two days for sprains and cold in the eyes. Use potency 30.

CHAPTER SEVEN

SYMPHYTUM OFFICINALE

Symphytum belongs to the Natural Order *Boraginaceae*, a small group which includes the familiar Myositis, or Forget-Me-Not. The Herbalists call it Comfrey, Bone-set, Consolida, or the Healing Herb. The plant grows to about two feet, with large rough leaves which can make the hands itch if handled. It has white or purple flowers growing on short stalks. The plant grows on river banks and ditches, and flowers in the early summer. Consolida says what the plant does. It consolidates and its name Comfrey, by which it is best known, is from the French *comfrie*.

Dr Fernie, in his *Herbal Simples,* relates how a locksmith at Teddington broke his little finger, which was painful and 'crunched'. A passing doctor said: 'You see that Comfrey growing there? Take a piece of its root and champ it, and put it about your finger and wrap it up.'

According to Dr Fernie the man did so and in four days his finger was well. Dr Clarke says: 'Symphytum may be considered the orthopaedic specific of herbal medicines and Dr Fernie's story confirms this'.

The first outstanding success I had with *Symphytum* happened in 1942 when I was called out to see a very old lady of ninety-five, who had been one of my earliest patients. She had been the wife of the Superintendent of Victoria Infirmary, Glasgow, and had fallen and sustained a Colles fracture of her right wrist. I wanted to send her into the hospital where her husband had reigned supreme, to have the wrist x-rayed and properly set. She would not hear of it and commanded me to set the wrist myself – a task which daunted me for I had never done such a job before.

I warned her that she might never be able to write again – and she conducted a voluminous correspondence – but none the less, she insisted that I set the wrist. I did the best I could, wrapped the wrist firmly in a bandage soaked in *Symphytum*, and left it on for six weeks, with instructions to soak the bandage in *Symphytum* every other day. When it was taken off the cosmetic result would not have pleased a surgeon, but the following Christmas she sent me a fine book with a dedication in her own shaky handwriting: 'To my dear doctor, who might have been a surgeon had he wanted to'. She died two years later but I am proud of that book to this day.

Incidentally, many homoeopathic patients reach their nineties, which is further proof of the safety and gentleness of our medicines.

The great Gerard published his immortal *Herball* in 1597 – the year Queen Anne was pleased to grant unto the said John Gerrard: 'One garden plot or piece of ground belonging to and adjoining on the east part to a mansion house called Somersett House in London'. Thus our first official herbal garden came into being at the rent of five shillings yearly. Of Comfrey, Gerard wrote:

The roots of Comfrey stamped, and the juice drunk with wine, helpeth those that spit blood and healeth all inward wounds and bursting, the same bruised and laid to in the manner of a plaister, doth heal all fresh and green wounds and are so glutinative, that it will solder and give together meat that is chopped in pieces, seething in a pot, and make it in one lump.

Gerard's idea of using Comfrey to solder together meat 'that is chopped up' might be taken up by careful housewives to eke out the left-overs in these hard times when even the price of mince is astronomical!

Dr Margery Blackie reports a case of a cyst on the jaw-bone operated on and which left a swelling on the cheek which disappeared after being treated by Comfrey.

TUMOUR DISAPPEARS

Sir William Thomson of Dublin, related in *The Lancet* (28/11/1896) a case of a man with a malignant tumour of the antrum, extending to the nose. It was a round-celled sarcoma. Operation was at first refused, but Thomson operated that year. A month later the growth began to show again, increased rapidly, closed the right eye, was blue, tense, firm, lobulated, but did not break. Thomson declined to operate again. Early in October – he had his operation in May – the patient walked into Thomson's surgery completely well. 'The tumour had completely disappeared from the face, and I could not identify any trace of it in the mouth'. The man had applied poultices of Comfrey root, and the swelling disappeared.

Dr Nash says that if a nerve is injured, *Hypericum* is the remedy, if the periosteum, *Ruta,* if the bone, *Calcarea Phos*. or *Symphytum*.

ARTHRITIC HIP

One of our most distinguished golf club makers lives in St Andrews. He is a large heavy man and had an arthritic hip which was operated on. The operation was not a success – perhaps due to the fact that this fine craftsman kept on working at his bench, making golf club heads for wooden clubs – heavy work, shaping persimmon and the toughest of hard woods. He is always in considerable pain, but a monthly dose of *Symphytum* has kept him at his employment for the last eighteen months, and the clubs he makes are second to none. I am the proud possessor of three, which I take in to be polished every few months, but he despairs of me, for I forget to put the covers on and he says they do not do him credit. He has now gone to have his hip replaced – a more modern operation.

In Mrs C.F. Leyel's fine book, *Cinque Foil*, she heads her first chapter 'Wound Herbs', listing thirty popular with herbalists. The first four on her list are Agrimony, Bugle, Cocklebur and Comfrey. Comfrey is the only one much used by homoeopaths, but I will consider Agrimony later, if only because it once figured in the London *Pharmacopoeia* as a wound salve.

Bugle or Bugleweed is known to us as *Lycopus Virginicus* of the National Order *Labiatae*. It has the homoeopathic reputation of gently lowering the blood-pressure. Mrs Leyel has a good word for Comfrey. She says: 'It heals both internally

and externally', which fact seems confirmed by
Sir William Thomson's Sarcoma case.

The second four in her list are Crosswort,
Daisy, Darnel, and Delphinium, of which Daisy
is important. Darnel (*Lolium Temulentum*) has
been proved, and used for intermittent
claudication, without much success. Her third
group of four are Dittany, Flax, *Arnica* (Leopards
Bane) and Madonna Lily. We have dealt with
Arnica. Flax mixed with lime water, was known
as Carron Oil, and was the popular treatment for
burns in my youth.

Thus we can say, out of the first three groups,
of Mrs Leyel's four wound herbs, we, as
homoeopaths, are grateful for three winners,
Symphytum, Bellis, and the great *Arnica* – all of
whose worth we have proved times without
number.

Of the others, Mrs Leyel lists: Marsh Mallow,
Matico, Medlar Mignonette, Moonwort,
Moneywort, Prunella, Rattles, Siegesbeckia,
Slippery Elm, Snowdrop, Spagnum Moss, Water
Soldier, Wood Sanicle, Wound Wort,
Ploughman's Spikenard which is our *Inula,* or
familiar *Scabwort*. I grow some in the garden. It has
large leaves and small purple flowers, and it is
supposed to be the herb Helen put in her corsage
when she ran off with Paris. It has a pleasant
aromatic smell, but as she was reputed to be so
desirable surely she had no need of this?

Inula is not a great homoeopathic medicine. It
has been tried in difficult cases of chronic
bronchitis, with disappointing results.

Two other familiar names in the list are
Slippery Elm and Spagnum Moss. Slippery Elm

is the Red Elm of America, and it gets its name
on account of the large amount of mucilage
contained in the inner bark. I had an old lady
once as a patient who ate the stuff like porridge
every morning, and claimed that it kept her
'comfortable'. She had what she called a 'nervous
stomach' and no appetite: as well as a food, it is
sold as a coarse powder to make into poultices,
and was once widely used for suppurations and
abscesses.

ANTI-DROUGHT MEASURE
When I was a lad during the First World War I
can recollect being sent out to gather Spagnum
Moss for the Red Cross. It holds water like a
sponge and was much used then for absorbent
bandages. As an anti-drought measure it might
be a good idea to have it cultivated around our
reservoirs, though in boglands in Scotland it is
apt to degenerate into peat.

Peat gets dearer and more popular for use by
amateur gardeners year after year – its only
virtues as I see it, is that it keeps down weeds and
holds moisture longer than soil can do.

I cannot finish this short study of *Symphytum*
without relating to you a true incident which
occurred in the practice in 1942 – in the grim
years of the black-out in Glasgow.

One of my patients, a lady of uncertain years,
most anxious to do her bit, was returning from
voluntary service at a hospital when she had a
motor accident in one of our dim streets. She
sustained a comminuted fracture of her left leg
and was in the Claremont Nursing Home, where
my surgeon brother-in-law had set it and I was

there with *Symphytum;* helping also to put on the plaster of Paris. The presiding genius of this home was Sister Mackie, who was a rather starchy, elderly lady, who was assisting in the theatre.

My brother-in-law was very tired. He had just returned from a visit to an air-raid shelter at Yarrow's shipbuilding-yard, which had received a direct hit, and where, against the advice of the air raid wardens, he had crawled in among the sagging concrete, and amputated the leg of a man who was trapped.

In the corridor outside the operating theatre of the home could be heard the steady sound of marching feet, walking up and down. This annoyed my surgeon brother-in-law, and also Sister Mackie, who asked me to investigate and get it stopped, for the home was full of many sick folk, and it was midnight.

I left the theatre, and there outside was a massive sergeant of the Seaforth Highlanders, in full uniform, striding up and down in his army boots. I asked him what the trouble was and he said he was worried – his wife was being delivered in the next room of her first baby by Sister Duncan. I said he was not to worry, Sister Duncan was expert at her job. 'It often happens to a husband that he gets worried, but it is a common experience'. 'That may be, sir,' said the Sergeant, 'but it's no that common when it happens while a chap is on his honeymoon.' This is a true story, which I related to Sister Mackie, but she was not amused. Both the baby and our patient made a good recovery.

It had been a wild night of Glasgow's worst

bombing, and when we got home, about 2 a.m. my younger sister said she had not been too worried. She had made up her bed under the dining-room table, and had felt quite safe!

NOTES ON DOSAGE

Keep a 5g stock of pills and give one every four hours each day for a week following fractures of neck of femur or wrist after bones have been pinned or set. It is also useful for black eyes. Use potency 30.

CHAPTER EIGHT

URTICA URENS

Urtica Urens is the lesser or small stinging nettle, used by homoeopaths in tincture form for first-degree burns, such as from a steaming kettle or hot stove. If applied at once it will prevent blisters forming.

The poet Thomas Campbell said in one of his letters: 'in Scotland I have eaten nettles, I have slept in nettle sheets, and dined off a nettle table-cloth. The young and tender nettle is an excellent pot herb. The stalks of the old nettle are a good as flax for making cloth. I have heard my mother say she thought nettle-cloth more durable than linen'.

Here is another quote from Dr D.M. Gibson:

In contact with the skin Urtica produces an acute burning sensation, followed by itching and local swelling. It was formerly thought that these toxic effects were caused by Formic Acid. More recent research has show that the nettle hair consists of a fine capillary tube calcified at its lower end, silicified at its upper end, and closed at the tip in the shape of a tiny bulb. This bulb breaks off when it comes in contact with the skin, leaving exposed a fine point. The pressure of contact drives this fine tube into the skin. The hair fluid contains high concentration of Histamine 0.1% and even higher concentrations of Acetylcholine (1%). In addition a third substance was found which contracts smooth muscle, but this has not been identified.

(*Homoeopathy*, Jan/Feb 1976)

If *Urtica* is kept in the family medical chest a drop or two applied to the sting of a bee gives relief at once, and if the patient complains that he is in for an attack of shingles, because he or she feels stinging pains, no matter if the pains are on the lips, the face, or beneath the breasts – a light application of *Urtica* tincture often prevents the herpes from developing.

SUPERFICIAL BURNS

Our main use for *Urtica* however, is for superficial burns – what we used to call burns of the first or second degree.

An old doctor told me once that when he was out for a walk he came across a caravan once where a man was applying compresses of cold tea to his wife's hand, which she had burnt with a recalcitrant primus stove. The caravan was attached to their car in a remote part of the Highlands beside a burn where there was a profusion of nettles beside a ruined cottage.

The doctor, a helpful and enterprising type, asked the man to boil a kettle for hot water. He then picked two handfuls of the nettles, put them in a pan and poured the boiling water over them. Taking two clean handkerchiefs, he placed them on the badly swollen hand, and poured the infusion on the linen. The pain went at once, and the couple were so grateful that the doctor got a free lunch, which the lady was able to prepare. It is an old gipsy remedy. Gipsies know a lot about country lore.

Another case I was told about – also in the far North – was when a gipsy came to a lonely cottage to see if they had brass candlesticks to sell

– (in the old days it was pots and pans they wanted, but now brass is a better market). The son of the house had been hit by his sister with a stick and had a real purler of a black eye. The gipsy took an over-ripe apple, cut it in two, and applied the cut surface to the eye with a firm bandage and next day the eye was back to normal.

TREATMENT OF GOUT

Urtica Urens has a long-established reputation in the treatment of gout – due to the enthusiasm of Dr Compton-Burnett, father of thirteen children, but of one outstanding one, Dame Ivy Compton-Burnett – a novelist whose literary work has been compared to Jane Austen and George Eliot. Personally, I think her novels are an acquired taste, but there is no doubt that her father, Dr James Compton-Burnett, was a name to conjure with in homoeopathic circles at the beginning of the century. He was an uncle of our own Dr Margery Blackie, who wrote *The Patient Not The Cure*, and who is the first lady doctor to hold the high appointment of personal physician to the Queen, a post she succeeded to from Sir John Weir, who was personal homoeopathic physician to four reigning monarchs.

Dr J. Compton-Burnett made a great reputation in curing many diseases but he will always be remembered for his revival of *Urtica* for gout. His routine prescription was to give five drops of the mother tincture of *Urtica* in a wine-glass of warm water, every two or three hours – it made the patient pass great quantities of gravel.

Now gout is a disease not often met with today.

It is a disturbance of purine metabolism, with an increase of uric acid in the blood, which leads to an attack of acute arthritis, and deposition of sodium biurate in and about the small joints – particularly the big toe joint, which can become intolerably tender. One reason why it is not so common is because claret and burgundy have become too expensive to be served each day, and the only ones who get gout have inherited the tendency from their fathers or grandfathers, who were martyrs to it, the sins of the fathers being visited on the children.

Dr Compton Burnett was fond of *Urtica Urens* and used it in the form of Nettle tea in all his cases of ague and malaria, often with good results. *Urtica* is one of these remedies whose outstanding modality is periodicity. There is a characteristic period recurrence of symptoms, which perhaps led the good doctor to use it for malaria.

NETTLES FOR VITAMIN C

Nettles are always found close to where there is, or was, human habitation. They are full of trace elements, which make them ideal for the compost heap. Nettles have always been a great favourite with herbalists to cleanse the blood, as a source of iron they exceed sorrel, and they are a good source of Vitamin C – better, some say, than rose-hip syrup. Nettle tea is a comfortable gargle for sore throats, and has long been a favourite with asthmatical and bronchial subjects.

Old Samuel Pepys liked nettle porridge, which is a mixture of young nettle leaves, dandelion leaves, watercress, sorrel leaves, blackcurrant leaves, a little mint or thyme, and one onion. Plenty of iron and Vitamin C in that lot but Scotsmen still prefer to stick to porridge made with oatmeal.

At the back of Audrey Wynne Hatfield's excellent little book *How To Enjoy Your Weeds* (Frederick Muller) – which my wife bought thinking it was a treatise on appreciating husbands – there are a couple of pages devoted to 'the weeds to relieve your aches, pains, boils and blames'. The author lists forty-two complaints out of which she suggests that the nettle is good for eleven of them; Anaemia, Asthma, Bladder disorders, Bronchial complaints, Colds, Gout, Gravel, Hair out of condition, Nettle rash, Rheumatism, Sore throat. Strangely enough the nettle takes second place to the dandelion, which she recommends thirteen times.

The dandelion is our *Taraxacum*, a homoeopathic remedy which I have used for mapped tongue, housemaid's knee and night sweats but without much success. Perhaps it should be re-proved, for I am one of those who think that all medicals should pay far more attention to herbal lore, where the accumulated knowledge of generations is available for all to study.

The weakness, as I see it, of herbal medicines is that in the old days, such plants as nettles and dandelions were used too often as panaceas for most of the ills to which our poor flesh is heir. Homoeopathy is more selective by our own peculiar method of modalities, but the allopaths would rather isolate the alkaloids from the plants and synthesize their own products, with the help

of the pharmaceutical manufacturers. Sometimes, alas, they bite off more than they can
chew, and the resulting product has side effects
past understanding.

NOTES ON DOSAGE

Every household should keep *Urtica* in stock in
'mother' tincture 4 fl. oz. (100 ml) and in pill form
(5g).

Apply 'mother' tincture diluted in equal part
with water for first degree burns, and use the pills
– one four times a day – for urticarias. Use
potency 30.

CHAPTER NINE

FIVE LESSER WOUND REMEDIES

ACONITE

This deadly poisonous plant, also known as *Monkshood* or *Wolfsbane,* has the reputation of being more poisonous to carnivora than to herbivora. It belongs to the Natural Order *Ranunculaceae* – 'The Little Frogs'; a large order which includes the greedy buttercups – whoever thought they resembled frogs?

Dr John H. Clarke states that *Aconite* is more closely associated with the rise and progress of homoeopathy than any other members of the Materia Medica.

Though one of the deadliest and most rapidly acting of poisons, through Hahnemann's method of attenuation in potencies above the third, it is a perfectly safe medicine at any age. It is not a great vulnerary or wound medicine except in one particular – it is one of our greatest medicines for relieving pain – the other two are *Chamomilla* and *Coffea* in potency. It relieves both pain and fear. The pains calling for *Aconite* are intolerable driving to desperation, the pains are tearing, cutting, are attended with restlessness, accompanied by numbness, tingling or formication (Clarke) and great anxiety.

Dr Tyler quotes a case of Sir John Weir's. He was called out to see a man suffering from Urticaria-Anaphylactic – after getting an injection of anti-tetanus serum. The patient was almost beside himself with fear and anxiety. He could not keep still. He was certain he was going to die. He got *Aconite* in the 30th potency and in fifteen minutes he was quite himself again.

APIS MELLIFICA

Though not strictly a wound healer, this is a remarkable homoeopathic medicine, tinctures of which can be made from the whole bee. It is also known as *Apis Virus*. The great Dr Hering wrote: 'There are different preparations of Apis but there is but one right one. It is the pure poison obtained by grasping the bee with small forceps, and catching the minute drop of virus suspended from the point of the sting in a vial or watch glass. This is then potentized'.

Dr Hering prescribed *Apis* for redness and swelling with stinging and burning pains; just what one would expect from a bee sting, with relief from cold compresses. *Apis* is a great throat medicine and especially good for children where the throat swells up, and where the uvula hangs down like a transparent sac full of water.

It is one of the remedies to be thought of in housemaid's knee where the knee is swollen, shiny, sensitive, sore and where there are the characteristic stinging pains. Dandelion (*Taraxacum*) is also given for housemaid's knee. *Apis* should also be remembered for painful styes about the eyes; it helps to prevent their recurrence, and several homoeopaths have recorded good results from *Apis* in high potency for arthritis in back and limbs. One of my favourite quotations is the following:

They are not worthy of the Honeycomb,
Who shun the hive because the bees have stings.

Nervous Bridegrooms

I use it when I encounter nervous bridegrooms who cannot make up their minds if they are 'doing the right thing'. Of course I give them *Argentum Nitricum*, potency 30, in addition. *Argenium Nit.* is Nitrate of Silver, and one of our best medicines for Anticipatory 'fears. It is a strange fact, but true, that in all my years in practice, I have encountered at least a dozen nervous bridegrooms, but never a nervous bride.

Old Pythagoras was fond of the classic maxim:

Whoever wishes to preserve his health should eat every morning before breakfast young onions with honey.

Sound advice, but a strange combination, though we homoeopaths use the red onion in potency to stop a running cold.

Mead is made from honey boiled with water, and exposed to the sun, after adding chopped raisins and lemon peel, and it was the Germans who had Myromel, or Honey wine – much the same as Mead – and they drank this for the first thirty days after marriage: hence the name honeymoon.

SILICA

Silicia, Silicon dioxide, pure flint, makes up the greater proportion of the earth's crust, and Silicates are taken up by plants and deposited on both the surface and interior of the stems.

Hahnemann introduced it into medicine by

his special method of attenuating insoluble substances. *Silicia* is the plant's corset, and keeps it upright – the strength of straw comes from *Silica*. Thus it follows that *Silica* types are easy to spot – a child needing[1] homoeopathic *Silica* usually lacks fibre – both physical and moral and wants support.

It is not a medicine however, for the lay public – usually following on *Pulsatilla* for the yielding youngster, who has not much resistance to disease. In low potencies it can be used successfully for whitlows, crops of boils and carbuncles, for it does help suppuration, and pus is better out than in. An examinee once wrote: 'Silica can let out puss.' But it is not so efficient as that!

Remedy for Bed-wetting
Equisetum – scouring rush, growing in damp soils, contains about 18 per cent *silica*. Many a mother has been grateful for it is a grand remedy for enuresis – bed-wetting – one of the great nuisances in nervy children in a large household, where washing bills increase year by year.

AGRIMONY
Agrimony has the botanical name *Agrimonia Eupatoria*, and belongs to the Natural Order *Rosacea*. *Agrimonia* comes from a Greek word and means 'shining', while the second word *Eupatoria*, refers to 'liver'.

The plant was supposed to help cataracts and liver complaints.

The plant has yellow blossoms from June to September, and it was John Gerard who wrote:

'A decoction of the leaves is good for them that have naughty livers'.

As far as I know, *Agrimony* has not been proved homoeopathically, but it is given here as one of the oldest of wound medicines. The herb formed part of the genuine Arguebusade water, as prepared against wounds inflicted by an Arquebus – an early type of portable gun – time has shot off the first letter, for the gun was once called Harquebus. It had a small calibre and could be fired through loop holes, and was popular in the sixteenth century.

A Useful Gargle

By pouring a pint of boiling water on a handful of the whole plant, stems, flowers, and leaves, it was possible to produce a useful gargle.

Agrimony was at one time listed in the London Materia Medica as a vulnerary herb. Nowadays perhaps that is its one substantial claim to fame, except for its use by herbalists. It is not a herb with which I am familiar.

Dr Boericke, on page 324 of his pocket Materia Medica, appears to think *Agrimonia* and *Cockleburr* are one and the same, though Mrs Leyel, usually accurate in such matters, lists *Cockleburr* as *Xanthium Spinosum*. Dr Fernie appears to agree with Boericke, and says *Agrimony* is also called *Cockelburr* or *Sticklewort*, because its seed vessels cling by the hooked ends of their stiff hairs to any person or animal coming in contact with the plant.

Pliny called *Agrimony* a plant of 'princely authoritie.'

Agrimony is not to be confused with *Hemp*

Agrimony, sometimes called *Rusticorum Panacea.* Its botanical name is *Eupatorium Cannabinum* of the Natural Order *Compositae.* It was once called 'Holy Rope' and was believed to be the hemp that bound Jesus to the Cross.

The hemp variety grows to a height of four or five feet with flower masses of dull lilac colour.

RHUS TOXICODENDRON

Rhus Tox. or Poison Ivy, is not one of our great injury remedies. It belongs to the Natural Order *Amacardiaceae,* which included our marking nut – one of our best medicines to think of when a patient complains her husband is getting into the habit of swearing at life and at her. It has the symptom of an intense itching eczema – which one could expect from poison ivy – but it also has that type of sudden lumbago and back pains which are better if the patient moves about and receives warm massage.

Back Pain

If the patient has been gardening and is seized with a sudden pain in his back and cannot bear movement, *Bryonia* – the wild hop of Germany, is the remedy to think of, especially if, once he gets to bed, he is morose and complains that the bed is too hard. If, however, the gardener's wife feels that her husband thinks that he is on his last legs, the thing she should do is to give him *Aconite,* and send for the family doctor.

Men are more dramatic about sudden pain than are women, a more stoical breed, who come to realize that suffering is the badge of all their tribe.

When I was very young, I had my first lesson in sudden back pains – an uncertain field of medicine. We lived a biscuit-throw from the local bowling green, to which my father went every Saturday. It was towards the end of the Great War, and my mother was having one of her many Red Cross meetings in the house that afternoon. She was not pleased with the overgrown privet-hedge, which she insisted my father cut before he went to bowls. He took a sudden back pain, got *Arnica*, and was made to finish the job.

About a month later we went through the same performance – the hedge had to be cut before the ladies came, and I was the boy to pick up the cuttings. Reluctantly my father started, when we were visited by an Irish tramp-like fellow. He said to my father: 'Your shears are blunt, Sir. For a matter of five shillings I will take them away and sharpen them'. The deal was made. We never saw either the tramp nor the shears again, but my father got his bowls without any back pains.

IMPORTANT WOUND REMEDIES

Dr Kent wrote that the surgery of homoeopathy largely involves the use of *Arnica, Rhus Toxicodendron, Ledum, Staphisagria, Calcareas,* and *Hypericum.* He says this in his lectures on Materia Medica, published in 1904. It is my opinion that in considering wound remedies, *Arnica, Ledum,* and *Hypericum* are the important ones and *Rhus Toxicondendrom, Calcareas* and *Staphisagria,* even in the field of surgery, are of minor importance. Dr Kent might have mentioned *Phosphorus,* which was a good antidote to chloroform in the old days.

I have mentioned very briefly the role of *Rhus Tox.*, and *Staphisagria* has a very useful part to play when sphincter muscles have been overstretched.

Dr Kent's remarks came in his lecture to the students on *Hypericum.* He finishes up by saying that when the patient is far gone, with cold breath, prostration, loss of blood, instead of giving *Carbo. Veg.* (our homoeopathic Corpse Reviver) he suggests *Strontia Carboniate. Arnica* is quite as efficient.

I could never see any occasion for using any of the Calcium salts in cases of surgery, but we must remember Dr Kent was lecturing when surgery was in a primitive state of development.

NOTES ON DOSAGE

Aconite. Keep a 5g stock of pills and give one every two hours at the start of a cold. Use potency 30.

Apis, Silica and *Agrimony*
These are all minor remedies and it is not absolutely necessary to stock them in the house.

Rhus Toxicodendron
It is well worth stocking a 5g bottle of pills for the sudden lumbago attack, when the patient has difficulty in moving but improves as he gets going about. Use potency 30.

CHAPTER TEN

CONSTANCY

Constancy is defined in the dictionary as the state or quality of being unmoved in mind; steadfastness, firmness, fortitude. Another definition is the quality of being invariable. Uniformity (Oxford Dictionary). Chambers Dictionary defines constancy as fixedness, or unchangeableness.

I like the shorter definition, though the quality I want to stress as regards homoeopathy is uniformity or unchangeableness. Some may like better the word consistency, which is defined as the quality, state or fact of being consistent, but constancy is the better word for our purpose.

To paraphrase John Bunyan (1628-1688):

He who would valiant be
'Gainst all disaster,
Let him in constancy
Follow the master.

If we think of the master as Hahnemann, that verse would be no bad motto to put above our Homoeopathic Hospitals. We stress the safety, the gentleness, the convenience, the cheapness, the certainty of our homoeopathic medicines, but we do not lay enough stress on consistency.

HOMOEOPATHS BELIEVE IN CONSTANCY

Constancy is one of the old-fashioned virtues. It is not held in high regard by people – look at the

ever increasing number of divorces; not by
pharmaceutical manufacturers – look how they
follow fashion in their products; nor is it followed
by the politicians, who change their policies,
trimming their sails to every wind that blows.
Homoeopaths – true homoeopaths – however,
believe in constancy, because their philosophy is
built on the sure foundation of certain basic laws
which never change.

These remarks are occasioned by my reading
an article in *The Times* on 1 September 1976. It
was headed 'Homoeopathic Medicine: an
alternative which deserves more than prejudice',
and it was written by Dr Margery Blackie,
Physician to the Queen since 1968.

It was a very good article, in which she
indicated that if the patient has a chest infection,
wants to lie on the affected side, and is very
thirsty, *Bryonia* is indicated; if he wants someone
near and needs reassurance, think of *Phosphorus*;
or if he wants to be alone and resents
disturbance, think of *Natrum Sulph*: or should he
want all the doors and windows open, ignoring
draughts, think of *Pulsatilla*.

Now these are simple examples of indications
for remedies known to every homoeopath,
practising anywhere in the world; and he would
be a poor homoeopath who did not latch on to
the remedy at once from the indications given.
This is what I mean by consistency. It is even
more apparent in a homoeopathic household. I
have seen youngsters of ten years of age going to
the homoeopathic medical chest after a fall or a
knock and taking an *Arnica* pilule, just as I have
seen others with cut fingers take *Calendula*

tincture and put a drop or two on a rag to wrap round the cut to stop the bleeding.

It is not so with allopathic medicine, where the latest thing advertised by the medical press is prescribed by the young doctor, anxious to impress the senior partner that he – the assistant – is at least keeping abreast of the times. He might not even be aware of what the patient got last time from the senior partner, unless the patient had been wise enough to keep the bottle containing the capsules. Even then the chemist's label may be illegible.

AN ANSWER TO CRITICS

Of course Constancy is not without its critics. We homoeopaths get criticized by some because we have made no dramatic discoveries such as the antibiotics, or the steroids, or the cobalt rays. I counter this by saying if one has a good, reliable, trouble-free car, why change it for the latest, most expensive model on the road? Then I tell them this true story:

One of my friends got a lift in a magnificent Rolls Royce when coming home from the golf club. The proud possessor was demonstrating all the gadgets, but all my friend wanted to do was to get rid of the ash from his cigarette. He was about to flick it out of the partly opened window, when the owner pressed a button and the window slid up and severed his forefinger at the top joint. That could be called a side effect. They can be serious with modern medicines, but not with homoeopathy – or old-fashioned cars.

Homoeopaths are quite aware of the enormous strides made by medical science in the last half-century. When I was a medical student, one of our rather cynical professors in his valedictory lecture, said that all we required to have on starting up in practice, was a stethoscope, a book of death certificates, and a waste-paper basket. Things have improved since then, and patients are living longer, and the National Health Service gets the credit for it.

This may be so, but patients have been known to live long after eighty, before the National Health Service came into being, and especially if they were treated by the gentle, certain, and undramatic remedies employed by us for nearly two hundred years.

PIONEERS IN HOMOEOPATHY

'He would valiant be' is a phrase worth pondering. One hundred years ago it took great courage for the pioneers in homoeopathy to stand out against the establishment of orthodox medicine, and some day I would like to write a short history of the men who manned the outposts, who got no encouragement from the academics, but who survived and prospered by merit alone.

One such was William Sharp, M.D., F.R.S., at one time senior surgeon to the Bradford Infirmary. His *Essays on Medicine* published by Leath and Ross in 1874, is a book well worth reading. Many people must have thought so, for it went in to at least ten editions. In this book Sir J.Y. Simpson, of chloroform fame, comes out of the arguments in a very bad light. He did more to hold back homoeopathy in Edinburgh than anyone else.

Let me finish this brief essay with a true story.

In 1932, my brother, the late Thomas Douglas Ross, bought a fine, old-fashioned house in Newton Place, Glasgow, which had formerly belonged to a distinguished professor of jurisprudence. This part of Glasgow was known as 'the valley of death,' for practically every house belonged to members of the medical profession.

The bathroom was at the top of the house, so while one was being put in on a more convenient floor, my brother and I went off to Lochmaddy to fish, and left the house in charge of our elderly parents. Unfortunately, while we were away, the workmen crossed an electric wire with an unknown gas pipe, and there was a fire on a Saturday morning, with two fire brigades at the house.

Quickly it was got under control, and my mother went out to get provisions. Two of Glasgow's most distinguished professors were talking on the terrace as she passed. One said, 'I hear number three has been bought by a homoeopath. Isn't it typical! Fire engines! They will do anything to advertise, will those homoeopaths!'

NO NEED TO ADVERTISE

My mother, a stranger to them, could on occasion assume the manners of a duchess. She stopped and said, 'Excuse me, but I overheard your remarks. My sons have been up fishing in the North for a week, the fire could not have been started by them. Homoeopaths do not require to advertise. Their patients, and the results, do that for them'. She never cared much for Newton

Place after that, and was glad to get back to her suburban home.

When my brother went off to the war the day after it started, my brother-in-law, Dr Tom Gordon, my younger sister and myself lived in the house. I was made the air-raid warden for the terrace of two dozen houses. Everyone had a basement and at a meeting of all the occupants, I put forward the idea that we should knock a passage through each basement house, so that, in the event of a direct hit, we could get exits, but our next door neighbour, a doctor's widow, would have none of it. She had a charming daughter who had just become a doctor, and the widow did not trust homoeopaths. Perhaps she was right, for I was not married then. Incidentally, her daughter became Lady Isobel Barnett, a name to conjure with in the world of television.

INDIVIDUALIZED TREATMENT

Prejudice dies hard, even among the nicest, and best educated of people. I used to think the profession disliked us because they imagined that we were poaching on their preserves, and taking their patients from them to their financial disadvantage. This reason should have disappeared with the advent of the National Health Service, since there is now no monetary competition involved. Allopaths still get paid for panel patients they seldom see, while having their load lightened by losing from their panels those chronically sick patients who prefer the individualized treatment provided by a homoeopath.

Nowadays the National Health Service is bedevilled by politics. The bureaucrats find homoeopathy an awkward corner to negotiate, because they believe in the old socialist dogma that all men are equal and should be treated on similar lines. It is difficult to see how the two schools of thought can be reconciled.

CHAPTER ELEVEN

ANIMAL HOMOEOPATHY

Homoeopathy has a lot to offer in the treatment of animals, and often the treatment is rewarding from the results obtained.

For years we had a couple of bitches, a miniature poodle called Zoë, and a long-haired dachshund which we called Lotta. Both had long pedigrees from the Kennel Club, and after a life of about 14 years they now lie buried in the Dog Cemetery at the bottom of our garden, beside the grave-stones of nine others, belonging to the original owner of the house.

Zoë was bowled over by a motor car at the age of four, just after we had left Gleneagles Hotel. She was much shaken and bruised but no bones broken. I had my case with me, so she got *Arnica* 30 at once, and when we got home, I bathed her scraped legs with a weak solution of *Calendula,* and she recovered – but hated motor cars thereafter.

Lotta was very healthy, needing no medicine but an occasional powder of *Cina* (worm seed). Like most Germans she was fond of her food, and she would steal Zoë's if she got the chance. When she over-ate she would retire to the rubbish dump – eat quantities of couch-grass and bishop's weed and promptly be very sick, and ready for another meal.

Years ago I had a lady patient in Kilmacolm who 'phoned me to say she had an outbreak of gastro-enteritis among her valuable stock of chinchillas. Two veterinary surgeons said the stock would have to be destroyed, but *Arsenicum album* (potency 12x) in their drinking water, saved the thirsty chinchillas.

Another patient I had bred Great Danes: magnificent dogs, as big as ponies and a joy to look at. One she was hoping to sell suddenly developed stiffness in the rear legs, worse when he got up, but which seemed to improve once he got going. On this symptom alone he got *Rhus Toxiconendrom* (12x) – six powders dry on the tongue, and in ten days' time. he won a prize at a dog show.

GOLDEN RETRIEVER'S RHEUMATISM

Another friend of mine had a clever Golden Retriever, who used to accompany us round the Old Course at St Andrews. I am never lucky enough to find a golf ball lost on that famous course, but Julie seldom came home with less than a dozen, ferreted out from the whins and gorse bushes. When she was about twelve her master used to tie her up on the seventh tee and collect her again on his way back at the thirteenth hole, because she had rheumatism in her legs which was worse for movement. I gave her *Bryonia* (12x) and for the next two years she was able to complete the round, getting an occasional powder at long intervals.

As I never charged for my animal medication I was surprised to get a parcel of golf balls one Christmas – tied up with scarlet ribbon, attached to which there was a card: 'With love from Julie'. Such a present is difficult to explain to one's wife!

During the war in Glasgow I went to fulfil an urgent call to a widow of advanced years suffering from chronic bronchitis. She was much as usual, full of complaints about the hardness of the times and the injustice of a government who had left her with but a single servant. However, she was more concerned about her canary, lying on its back in the cage, and apparently breathing his last.

My patient had an old-fashioned fountain pen filler handy, so I put some *Carbo-Veg* (Vegetable Charcoal, potency 30), into a glass of water, stirred it up, and dropped a drop or two into the bird's open beak. By the time I had listened to the patient's numerous complains the bird was back on its perch singing lustily. This impressed the old girl far more than any attention I had been able to give her, and when I sent her my modest quarter's fee, she sent me a cheque for double that amount. I eased my conscience by bringing my friend, the canary, some chick-weed from the garden on subsequent visits.

BORAX FOR FOOT-AND-MOUTH

My greatest triumph in animal husbandry however happened towards the end of 1967 when there was a serious outbreak of foot-and-mouth disease in Cheshire and Shropshire. Six years before . I had written an article in our magazine *Homoeopathy* called 'Is the Slaughter Really Necessary?' (Dr Blackie refers to it in her book) and I suggested that *Borax* might be given as a prophylactic. About 100 farmers took up the suggestion and in those who did not have mixed farms – cattle and sheep –.we had much success.

One Friday I came back very tired from Glasgow after a hard week's work, to find a clutter of television vans and about a dozen people standing at my front door. They had been there all afternoon and wanted an interview. All I wanted was my dinner, so I sent them about their business. None the less, on the Sunday there was a long article in the *Scottish Sunday Express* complete with an awful photograph of myself. The article was headed 'Borax Has Saved Our Cattle Say 100 Farmers'.

Nelson's of London sent out at least a quarter of a million packets of *Borax* to the farmers, but the whole thing cost me money in long-distance phone calls and postage for replies to farmers asking for details, and could I suggest something for their wives and children, who were desolate and on the verge of nervous breakdowns, because every farm smitten had no life stirring. All animals had been slaughtered in the farms affected round about them and they were afraid they would suffer the same fate.

I chose *Borax* as a prophylactic for foot-and-mouth disease, because it has as a symptom, Aphthae about the mouth, and blisters about the feet, and the cow has a great dread of downwards motion – watch a farmer trying to coax a cow out of a float. Up in the Far North where the crofter may have two acres and a cow, the cow is part of the family. In the wet autumn if the cow picks up blisters about the feet the crofter would remove it to dry ground high up among the heather. The beast would get thin and listless, but in time would recover.

I have had several cases of farmers' wives

complaining that the hens were pecking at their eggs. For this I gave *Sepia* (the juice of the cuttle fish) with varying success. Once on the Ayrshire coast a Clydesdale mare had difficulty in dropping her foal. I was visiting the old farmer at the time, and the mare got *Caulophyllum* (30) in her drinking water, and she had a successful delivery. I was rewarded by Mr Howie giving the offspring my name.

Sepia is a female remedy with the mental characteristic – 'Indifference to those they love best.' Perhaps an odd choice for the hens but maybe they did not want chickens!

SHETLAND PONIES

Another patient of mine was a purser on one of the liners trading with America. He came from the far North and did a smart sideline in Shetland ponies, often taking over six at a time for the pampered children of the wealthy. The ponies were bad sailors, so the purser always had a supply of *Cocculus* to put in their drinking water, which seemed to work well.

Caulophyllum (Blue Cohash) is the squaw root of the old North American Indians, and it really does relax the muscles of reproduction. If it was used more often in midwifery there would be far less need of forceps deliveries or suction.

Cocculus (Indian Cockle) is a good remedy for sea sickness, car sickness and air sickness, and spasm of muscles, such as the ponies had in confined space, after a childhood of roaming free on the moors.

No doubt some veterinary surgeons will think the above a lot of nonsense. One said to me,

'Homoepathy as I understand it, is individual treatment. You prescribe on the symptoms alone, which you match to the symptoms listed for the drug. How can you do that with a dog or a cow?' I answered: 'Sometimes we get our best results with very young children and with animals. True, they cannot give a list of their symptoms, but we can observe and ponder what is required, if we have good knowledge of our drugs'.

As Dr Ronald Livingston remarks in *Homoeopathy – Born 1810 – Still Going Strong* (Asher Asher Press, 1973) – one of the most concise books written on the subject:

> Veterinary Homoeopaths, using the same approach, achieve similar and even more spectacular effects by relying on their imagination of what the suffering animal must be feeling. These improved results arise, in my opinion, from the simple fact that animals, unlike human patients, cannot dissimulate their feelings ... the only practical difference is that they speak what is to us a wordless language.

That could not be better expressed ... anyone seeing my Dachshund, Lotta, coming in to the consulting room with her large, sorrowful, liquid, eloquent eyes, full of repentance, would know that she had pinched Zoë's dinner, and that it was time for me to let her out of the French window. Down she would creep to the rubbish dump, eat the weeds, and come back perky as ever.

I am very glad the Faculty of Homoeopathy has opened its doors to the veterinary surgeons, with Mr McLeod's pioneer work; it should be a rewarding exercise for all concerned.

GLOSSARY

Homoeopathy
From the Greek words *homois,* meaning similar, and *pathos,* meaning suffering.

Modalities
Lists of aggravations or ameliorations (modifying influences) influencing the choice of the remedy. For instance, patients whose complaints are aggravated by cold generally require *Arsenicum, Calcium Carbonate, China, Kali. Carb., Nux Vomica, Phosphorus, Sepia,* while patients who cannot stand the heat are in a smaller group and may require *Apis, Argentum Nit., Natrum Mur., Pulsatilla* or *Sulphur.*

Potency
Not a fundamental part of homoeopathic philosophy, but the result of Hahnemann's practical experience. By the result of repeated dilutions and shakings he found that he released unsuspected power or, as he called them, dynamizations in the substance. Nowadays this is done by electrical mechanical shakings. Two scales are used, the decimal and the centesimal. From the mother tincture one drop is taken and diluted with nine drops of distilled water and alcohol and shaken many times in a clean test tube. This gives 1x, 1/10th concentration (10%). Using the diluted solution this process is repeated to achieve a potency of 2x, 1/100th

concentration (1%). The same is repeated for a potency of 3x, 1/1000th concentration (0.1%), and again for 4x, 1/10000th concentration (0.01%). On the more common centesimal scale 1c = 1/100th concentration (1%); 2c = 1/10000th concentration (0.01%); 3c = 1/1000000th concentration (0.0001%); 30c = 100^{30} concentration. Dilutions have been made to 50,000 in terms of the centesimal scale and even higher so that no trace of the molecule is seen or can be proved. The x (or in some countries D) must always be shown in decimal potencies, but in centesimal potencies the c is usually omitted.

Remedy
This is said to have been proved when an attenuated amount given to healthy persons brings on similar symptoms to the patient's complaints.

Repertory
A compilation of all the useful symptoms recorded in the Homoeopathic Materia Medica. The best, and most complete one, was compiled by J.T. Kent, A.M., M.D. and runs to 1493 pages. William Boericke, M.D., compiled a pocket manual of Homoeopathic Materia Medica, comprising the characteristic and guiding symptoms of all remedies.

Similia Similibus Curantur
Like cures like.

Types
Homoeopaths consider mental symptoms important. They get used to classifying their patients according to the characteristics of the

remedies. For instance, the *Arsenic type* is careful and tidy about his person and his home, while the *Sulphur type* is the exact opposite; the ragged philosopher in an untidy house. The *Lycopodium type* is the worried executive – grey-haired and with a deeply lined face. The *Pulsatilla type* is the weepy blonde, but the *Natrum Mur type* is the joyless female. The *Arnica type* wants to be left alone, cannot bear to be touched, and is indifferent.

USEFUL ADDRESSES
Homoeopathic Hospitals
The following provide facilities within the National Health Service:

The Royal London Homoeopathic Hospital, Great Ormond Street, London WC1N 3HR (Tel. 01-837 3091)

The Liverpool Homoeopathic Hospital 42 Hope Street, Liverpool L1 9DB (Tel. 051-709 8474)

The Bristol Homoeopathic Hospital, Cotham Road, Cotham, Bristol BS6 6JU (0272 33068)

The Glasgow Homoeopathic Hospital, 1000 Great Western Road, Glasgow G12 0NR (041-339 0382)
  Outpatients Department,
  5 Lynedoch Crescent, Glasgow G3 6EQ
  (041-332 4490)

Tunbridge Wells Homoeopathic Hospital, Church Road, Tunbridge Wells, Kent (0892 25065)

Homoeopathic Clinics

Surgeries are held by homoeopathic doctors at the following clinics, but it is necessary to telephone for an appointment:

Bath – at Belmont, Lansdown Road,
(Tel. 0225 4043)

Bradford – Monthly at 11 Heaton Grove, Frizinghill
(Tel. Bradford 44104)

Channel Islands – Monthly at St Matthew's Vicarage,
Millbrook, Jersey.
(Tel. Central 20934)

Essex – Thursday afternoons at The Surgery, Queen's Road, Earls Colne, Nr Colchester.
(Tel. Earls Colne 2022)

Isle of Wight – Periodically at 29 Victoria Avenue,
Shanklin.
(Tel. Shanklin 2306)

Leeds – Fortnightly on Wednesdays (2.30 to 5.30pm) at
30 Grove Road, Leeds 6.
(Tel. Leeds 757917)

London – Wednesday mornings (11.00 to 12.30) at
386 Upper Richmond Road West, Putney, London SW14 (Tel. 01-878 3512)

Manchester – Daily at Brunswick Street, Ardwick.
(Tel. 061-273 2446)

Surrey – Monthly at The Beeches, Wych Hill, Working, Surrey
(Tel. 048-62 61442)

Sussex – Most Tuesdays at 162 Goring Road, West Worthing.
(Tel. Worthing 46179)

Homoeopathic Chemists

A. Nelson and Co., 73 Duke Street, London W1M 6BY
(Tel. 01-629 3118)

H. Gould and Son, 67 Moorgate, London EC2
(Tel. 01-606 5359)

Kilburn Chemists Ltd., 211 Belsize Road, London NW6
(Tel. 01-328 1030)

Stewarts Pharmacy, 59 Sheen Lane, London SW14
(Tel. 01-876 1861)

John Biles, Galen Pharmacy, 1 South Terrace, South Street, Dorchester, Dorset
(Tel. 0305 3996)

Martins the Chemist, Goring Road, Worthing, Sussex

Weleda (UK) Ltd., Ship Street, East Grinstead, Sussex
(Tel. 010342 25933)

Renfrewshire Pharmaceuticals, 12 Lamgrig Road, Newton Mearns, Glasgow G77 5AA
(Tel. 041-639 4256)